About the authors

Gillian Rowe is a writer and researcher who has edited and authored the primary textbook for nursing associates. She has extensive experience in the health and social care sectors, in both nursing and managing residential care settings. She is a qualified lecturer, lecturing for University of Plymouth Partnerships, and delivers mental health training to the wider community. Gillian is an Associate Fellow of the Higher Education Academy.

Deborah Gee is a Senior Lecturer and Course Lead for the Specialist Community Public Health Nursing course (SCPHN) at Teesside University. In 2006, Deborah qualified as a registered nurse and has worked within a variety of settings, including Neonatal Intensive Care and Community District Nursing. In 2010, Deborah completed her PGDip SCPHN qualification and has significant experience working with families and young children, and assessing and identifying their health needs, and those of the wider population, in her role as a health visitor. Deborah has an MSc in Education in Professional Practice; she is a Fellow of the Higher Education Academy, in addition to holding recognised teacher status with the Nursing and Midwifery Council.

Ami Jackson began her nursing career as a cadet nurse and then completed her pre-registration training at Northumbria University in 2007. She then completed a Practice Development degree in 2013. Ami has worked in a variety of areas including stroke rehabilitation, acute older persons' medicine, intensive care and orthopaedic surgery. Ami became a ward sister on an orthopaedic trauma unit and developed significant experience in leadership and management. More recently, Ami was a Practice Placement Facilitator, leading on pre-registration nursing programmes within her local NHS Trust. Ami now tutors Training Nursing Associates at Teesside University, and has commenced a master's degree in Global Leadership.

Acknowledgements

The authors would like to thank Eleanor Rivers and Laura Walmsley for their invaluable support and advice during the writing of this book.

Our especial thanks go to John Wheatley and Dani Nash.

We would also like to thank our nursing associates for their contribution: Beth Parker and Angie Blakey.

The authors give love and thanks to their families and friends for their support during the writing process. We really could not have done it without you.

We are particularly grateful to Delores Campanario at the World Health Organization for permission to use WHO images, and to Charlene Burin for use of Sage images.

We dedicate this book to those we loved (and still love) who are no longer with us.

$$(\partial + m)\, \psi = 0$$

Introduction

About this book/Who is this book for?

This book has been written mainly for training nursing associates, but it contains information relevant for healthcare practitioners and social care workers. The book addresses the academic and practice skills you need to support the care you will give to your patients and clients both in settings and the community. As a qualified nursing associate within health and social care, you will actively engage with public health issues and tackling some of the inequalities experienced by individuals, populations and communities. The contents of this book will also support qualified nursing associates on the revalidation journey. This book will also provide an evidence-based guide for apprentice nursing associate's practice supervisors, academics and educators, and practice development nurses and clinical leads who supervise trainee nursing associates.

Why is *Health Promotion for Nursing Associates* the title of the book?

This book will focus on the underpinning theories that support the delivery of health promotion activities which are part and parcel of your care practice. It will support your professional formation and enhance your professional identity within your working environments. You will practice within multidisciplinary teams, working with patients across their lifespan and in specialist areas such as working with adults, children, those with poor mental health and those with learning disabilities. Once qualified, your role will require you to deliver safe, effective, responsive care in an ethical, non-judgmental manner. Gaining an understanding of the social determinants of health, health inequality and barriers to access to health will help you to support your patients to take control of their health.

Book structure

This book is divided into eight easy-to-read chapters. Although each chapter is standalone, there are links within the chapters that relate to similar further information on a topic in other chapters.

Chapter 1

This chapter introduces you to the underpinning principles and theoretical basis of health promotion. You will study health promotion models and consider how they relate to your practice. This chapter will help you to understand the complexities and challenges within notions of health and wellbeing.

Chapter 2

Here we focus on your communication skills. This chapter will explain the anatomy and physiology of hearing, speaking and cognition, and how they work together for communication. It will also consider your interpersonal skills, and how they can support you to become a behaviour change agent. This chapter also incorporates the voice of nursing associates and their 'lived experience', and will offer you the opportunity to examine how other nursing associates developed and practised their skills as a means to enhance your own development.

Chapter 3

This chapter explores the factors that lead to health inequalities. It examines how inequalities are measured and reported within society in order to inform healthcare provision and to target areas of need. We discuss how unequal differences within society can influence the health and wellbeing of individuals, especially vulnerable groups. You will use the knowledge you gain within this chapter to understand how inequality affects communities and populations.

Chapter 4

Here you will gain an understanding of early childhood and adolescence. We begin by examining the stages of brain development from birth to adolescence. Then we examine the importance of early childhood development and attachment. You will be introduced to the theories of attachment styles, and why they can have an impact across the lifespan. You will also consider the factors that influence healthy childhood development. Finally, you are asked to critically examine the current key priorities in public health.

Chapter 5

Chapter 5 provides an overview of the UK history of public health and infection prevention. We will then take an in-depth examination of Personal Protective Equipment (PPE) and antimicrobial stewardship, as well as its especial relevance in the time of Covid-19. We discuss the chain of infection and sepsis. We will also consider the legal framework that governs the safe handling of contaminated material and safe food hygiene in various settings.

Chapter 6

This chapter will discuss how we promote healthy lifestyles, introduce you to the theoretical models and give you guidance in their application. It will then go on to consider what making every contact count (MECC) is, and, equally importantly, what MECC is not, as defined by Health Education England (HEE). We will think about motivational interviewing and how to confidently start potentially difficult conversations with people. We will also examine some of the factors that behaviour change addresses, by studying the causes and health outcomes of poor lifestyle choices.

Chapter 7

This chapter will introduce you to some fundamental theoretical knowledge of mental health. We will consider notions of stigma, prejudice and stereotyping, and how these impact on individuals and their families. We will examine the underpinning theories of mental health then go on to discover the legal and ethical considerations that underpin care delivery. We will debate how mental health conditions are classified and why this is a source of contention. Finally, we will examine mental health promoting activities for both the people you will work with and for yourself.

Chapter 8

This chapter concerns data and demographics. Here, we explore the principles of epidemiology and examine what demography and population means in a health context. We will discuss using electronic data capture in public health, and look at how novel integrated medical devices are changing the delivery of healthcare to populations. We will consider health screening and vaccinations, something particularly relevant within the Covid-19 landscape. We will discuss how digital technology can be used to promote healthy lifestyles for individuals and specific groups.

Requirements for the NMC

The standards of proficiency represented within this book match the standards of knowledge and skills that a nursing associate will need to meet in order to be considered by the Nursing and Midwifery Council (NMC) as capable of safe and effective nursing associate practice. These standards have been designed to apply across all health and care settings, i.e., mental health, children's, learning disability and adult nursing. The chapters of this book are guided by the latest standards for nursing associates. The NMC (2018) *Standards of Proficiency for Nursing Associates* can be found at www.nmc.org.uk/standards/standards-for-nursing-associates/

Learning features

Learning from reading text is not always easy. Therefore, to provide variety and to assist with the development of independent learning skills and the application of theory to practice, this book contains activities, case studies, scenarios, further reading, useful websites and other materials to enable you to participate in your own learning. You will need to develop your own study skills and 'learn how to learn' to get the best from the material. The book cannot provide all the answers – but instead it provides a framework for your learning.

The activities in the book will, in particular, help you to make sense of, and learn about, the material being presented. Some activities ask you to reflect on aspects of practice, or your experience of it, or the people or situations you encounter. *Reflection* is an essential skill in nursing, and it helps you understand the world around you and often to identify how things might be improved. Other activities will help you develop key graduate skills, such as your ability to *think critically* about a topic in order to challenge received wisdom, or your ability to *research a topic and find appropriate information and evidence,* and to be able to *make decisions* using that evidence in situations that are often difficult and time pressured. Communication and working as part of a team are core to all nursing practice, and some activities will ask you to carry out *teamwork activities* or think about your *communication skills* to help develop these. Finally, as a registered nursing associate, you will be expected to *manage* your own case load or area of care, and so some activities focus on helping you build confidence in doing this.

All the activities require you to take a break from reading the text, think through the issues presented and carry out some independent study, possibly using the internet. Where appropriate, there are sample answers presented at the end of each chapter, and these will help you to understand more fully your own reflections and independent study. Remember, academic study will always require independent work; attending lectures will never be enough to be successful on your programme, and these activities will help to deepen your knowledge and understanding of the issues under scrutiny, and give you practice at working on your own.

You might want to think about completing these activities as part of your personal development plan (PDP) or portfolio. After completing an activity, write it up in your PDP or portfolio in a section devoted to that particular skill, then look back over time to see how far you are developing. You can also do more of the activities for a key skill that you have identified a weakness in, which will help build your skill and confidence in this area.

This book also contains a glossary on page 161 to assist you with unfamiliar terms. Glossary terms are in bold in the first instance that they appear.

We hope you enjoy reading this book and engaging in the activities. It will support your learning through your college course or apprenticeship, and again at revalidation. Supporting people to make healthy changes is one of the most life enhancing things you can do for your patients. Good luck with your studies and your future career.

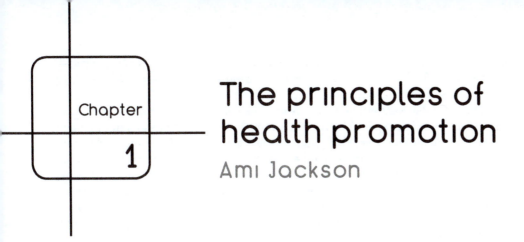

The principles of health promotion

Ami Jackson

Chapter aims

After reading this chapter, you will be able to:

1.   discuss notions of health and wellbeing;
2.   understand the principles of health promotion;
3.   explain the theoretical models of health promotion across the life span;
4.   navigate the complexities of health promotion and be able to apply this in practice.

Introduction

This chapter will examine the origins of health promotion and consider what health promotion is and how it is done. We will examine and discuss various health promotion models and compare their elements. We will also consider health promotion through the lifespan and examine health promotion and mental health. As you work your way through the chapter, there are opportunities to engage in activities to help you reflect on your practice. 'Health is, therefore, seen as a resource for everyday life, not the objective of living' (WHO, 1986).

The first 50 years of the twentieth century were drenched in the blood of the First and Second World Wars. At the end of the Second World War, people had had enough and wanted a better world. Many global organisations were born from this desire, one of which was the World Health Organization (WHO). The WHO promoted the idea that health was a human right, and not something for the privileged wealthy few. They wrote their definition of health as being 'not merely the absence of disease, but a state of complete physical, mental, spiritual and social wellbeing'. Many argued that this statement was unachievable or utopian. So, in 1986, in Ottawa, Canada, the first International Conference on Health Promotion formulated the following statement to create an understanding from a health promotion perspective.

Health promotion is the process of enabling people to increase control over, and to improve, their health. To reach a state of complete physical, mental, and social well-being, an individual or group must be able to identify and to realize aspirations, to satisfy needs, and to change or cope with the environment. Health is, therefore, seen as a resource for everyday life, not the objective of living. Health is a positive concept emphasizing social and personal resources, as well as physical capacities. Therefore, health promotion is not just the responsibility of the health sector but goes beyond healthy life-styles to well-being.

(WHO, 1986)

The *Ottawa Charter* is considered to be 'holistic' which means it takes into account spiritual, mental and social factors, rather than just the physical symptoms of a disease. The NMC (2018) draws on these themes in its assertion of the role that nursing associates play in health promotion.

Nursing associates play a role in supporting people to improve and maintain their mental, physical, behavioural health and wellbeing. They are actively involved in the prevention of and protection against disease and ill health, and engage in public health, community development, and in the reduction of health inequalities.

(NMC, 2018)

As described above, health promotion is the process of enabling people to increase control over, and to improve, their health. It moves beyond a focus on individual behaviour towards a wide range of social and environmental interventions (WHO, 2020b). Scott and Western (1998) recognised that the medical model is most frequently used when assessing individuals. It is disease-focused and is scientific in its approach. However, they point out that this is in strong contrast to the accepted ideology that the *Ottawa Charter* provides.

The *Ottawa Charter* (1986) identifies five action areas and three strategic areas for health promotion. It was the first charter for health promotion to address a global audience with the principles of health promotion. Let us first consider the five action areas, as shown in Figure 1.1.

The five action areas

1. *Building health and public policy*: Create policy that helps protect the health of individuals and the communities in which they live, in order to help individuals to make healthier choices. A synchronised approach is needed, so this includes legislative, regulatory and organisational efforts. For instance, promoting health in the workplace might include forming healthy eating groups or a walking group.

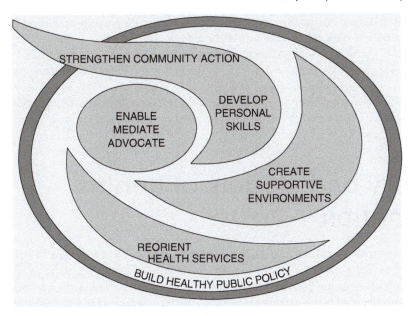

Figure 1.1 Building public health policy: The 5 action areas © WHO

Health policies are not created just for health departments, they are collaborative with other sectors such as local councils, government and charities.

2. *Creating supportive environments*: The environments in which individuals live are closely linked to their health. This element focuses on communities themselves, where individuals live, work or play. Enabling people to make health promoting choices is vital.
3. *Strengthening community action*: This means encouraging the collective efforts of communities to improve their health. Ever heard of the saying 'strength in numbers'? It can sometimes take just one person to make a small change that encourages others to follow. This could be community lunch groups supporting specific health education activities. Another example could be inviting diabetes awareness outreach workers to give a talk to a community group or workplace.
4. *Re-orientating health services*: Health services were traditionally medically focused on the curative treatment needs of individuals. The *Ottawa Charter* (WHO, 1986) considers that refocusing on people in their communities is taking a more holistic approach to health promotion. The *Ottawa Charter* also indicates that strengthening protective factors, reducing risk factors and improving health determinants will improve the health of people globally. This can be achieved by introducing community health educator roles.
5. *Developing personal skills*: This means developing social and life skills, in tandem with information education, in order to make positive health choices. Good examples of this are online educational programmes, weight management classes and clubs and giving information leaflets in community settings, such as pharmacies.

Having looked at the action areas, now let us look at the three strategic areas.

1. *Advocate*: This means using individual and political commitments, policy support and social actions to support a health goal.
2. *Mediate*: This is the process of uniting the statutory, private and voluntary sectors within communities, to reconcile them in ways that promote and protect health. Examples here

include NHS mental health services, private sector employers providing Improving Access to Psychological Therapies (IAPT), and the charity Mind.

3. *Enable*: In partnership with individuals, we need to empower people to engage in activities that will improve their health, such as joining an arts therapy group or exercise classes.

While the charter sets out clear actions regarding the importance of health promotion, we must ask ourselves how these evolved. To do this we need to understand the underlying theory of health promotion.

Theory and models of health promotion

The *Ottawa Charter* (1986) highlights key messages in relation to actions and strategies, as we have discussed, in order for people to reach their ultimate health goals. However, what are the fundamental elements of health? The areas are categorised into physical, mental and social wellbeing. It is imperative the individual identifies their own aspirations and sets out clear goals to achieve this, with both a health professional's support and the support of others around them.

Naidoo and Wills (2016) state that 'Health is a broad concept which can embody a huge range of meanings'. The authors discuss how people's perceptions are formed as to what 'good health looks like'. For example, you may have certain views on what health promotion is for you, due to your own life experiences, this may be influenced by your social class or education. Naidoo and Wills (2016) refer to this as 'lay' concepts of health. Lay concepts have developed through the social constructs you have been exposed to within your home, community and society. The authors note that there are many different beliefs within communities, and they may have different notions of what constitutes health. Examine Activity 1.1 and consider your own cultural beliefs for health protection. The activity asks you to compare your previous beliefs and your current beliefs. Has anything changed or have your beliefs been reinforced?

Activity 1.1   Reflection

What were the lay concepts of health that you were brought up with? Some lay health beliefs are entirely sensible and reasonable, while others have little basis in evidence or reality. These encompass family and community wisdom, such as eating sugar to get rid of hiccups, or taking honey and lemon when you have a cold.

What beliefs were you told would protect your health?

Reflect on your cultural health beliefs and compare them with the academic and theoretical knowledge you have now. What do you still believe and what has been discarded?

As this answer is based on your own reflections, there is no outline answer at the end of the chapter.

As you can see in your responses to Activity 1.1, we all have personal experience of lay explanations of health with our personal lay referral structure. Case Study 1.1 explores what this structure might look like, showing how we often consult a number of different people and authorities within our lives before turning to a health professional.

Case study 1.1 Applying the theory

After a night out with friends, Nish wakes up feeling unwell. He has a headache and an upset tummy, so he considers likely causes:

'Probably the curry and beer I had last night'.

Self-explanation

When Nish's symptoms do not go away after 12 hours, he asks his Mum and Nan for advice.

Family authority

His Mum and Nan discuss this and then suggest there is probably a bug going around, and he may have picked it up from one of his friends. Nish rings his friends to find out if they are okay. He describes his symptoms to his friend Jake, who says, 'Oh yes, Yasmin had that, she was proper poorly, but it went away after about a week'.

Circle of intimates

The following day, Nish's tummy feels better but he has started coughing and sneezing. His nextdoor neighbour has popped in for coffee and a chat and tells Nish that the local radio weather forecast says the pollen count is really high, and this might account for his sneezing.

Community authority

Only after the symptoms fail to clear within an expected time, or if they increase in severity, is a health professional consulted. This could be considered as a hierarchy of authority and drawn as a pyramid.

Health beliefs can be formed by cultural, historical and local influences, also emotional and behavioural factors. Recent emphasis centres on a personal individual responsibility model, but the above case study and an examination of your own beliefs leads us to consider that there are many more factors to health than just 'looking after yourself'. Therefore, we shall examine the dimensions that also feature in the *Ottawa Charter*.

As you can see from Figure 1.2, there are four interacting dimensions of holistic care and thus we should consider *physical health, psychological health, spiritual health* and *social health*. As professionals, we must examine the distinct influences and connections between them.

1. *Physical health*: focuses on the body: its anatomical and physiological state.
2. *Psychological/mental health*: focuses on a person's psychological and emotional wellbeing.
3. *Spiritual health*: recognises moral or religious principles or beliefs that bring peace to individuals.
4. *Social health*: refers both to a distinctive characteristic of society, and of individuals themselves.

Health Education England (HEE, 2020) states 'Being person-centred is about focusing care on the needs of [the] individual. Ensuring that people's preferences, needs, and values guide clinical decisions, and providing care that is respectful of and responsive to them'. The care we deliver to individuals should always be holistic and patient-centred and should not assume that the apparent physical symptoms are the sole root cause of illness.

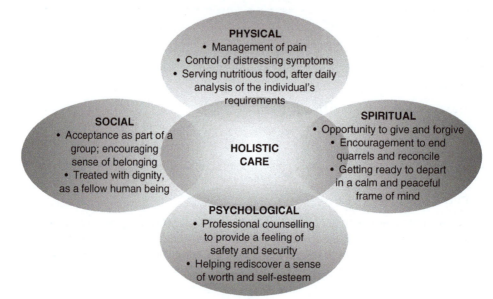

Figure 1.2   Holistic care

Maslow's (1943) work on the theory of human motivation indicates that an individual's actions are focused on the direction of goal achievement. Maslow encapsulates the essence of what human beings need to survive (see Figure 1.3). For example, going out with friends for a meal in a restaurant satisfies an individual's physiological needs, however, it also meets belonginess and love needs, which enhances wellbeing. This was something we all missed during the time of the Covid-19 **pandemic**, with many of us feeling the desire to be with loved ones and friends, and for life to get back to normal.

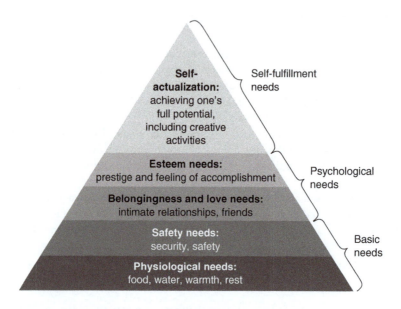

Figure 1.3   Maslow's hierarchy of needs (1943)

Wellbeing can be defined as how people feel and function, not only on a personal level but socially too. NHS (2019b) states there are five steps to wellbeing:

1. connect with other people;
2. be physically active;
3. learn new skills;
4. give to others;
5. pay attention to the present moment (mindfulness).

Pike and Forster (1995) identified that health promotion is delivered within the context of ongoing change. We must take into consideration other factors that relate to health promotion. In the next section, we introduce the concept of the determinants of health, which are further developed in Chapter 3.

Determinants of health

The concept of the determinants of health are not only about individuals but of populations too. Marmot et al. (2020) explain that people living in different socio-economic environments face different risks of ill health and even death. For example, those in a higher social class have a greater life expectancy.

Determinants of health are variable between individuals and across population groups in terms of life expectancy and health outcomes. To understand the determinants of health, we must first address the factors that influence health. Factors that influence a person's health include those that are more fixed, such as age, sex and genetic factors. They also include the good or poor health behaviours people engage in, such as smoking, excessive alcohol intake, physical activity and diet. Health is also influenced by the conditions people are born into, work, live and grow up in. This includes their social networks, socio-economic status, cultural, environmental state and the health systems they can access. Collectively, these factors are called the social determinants of health (WHO, 2020b) and are helpfully illustrated in Dahlgren and Whitehead's (1991) 'policy rainbow' which you can see in Figure 1.4.

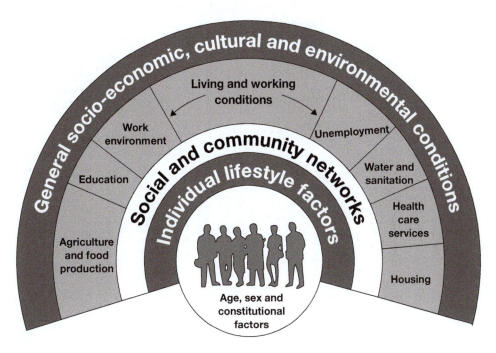

Figure 1.4 Dahlgren and Whitehead, social determinants of health

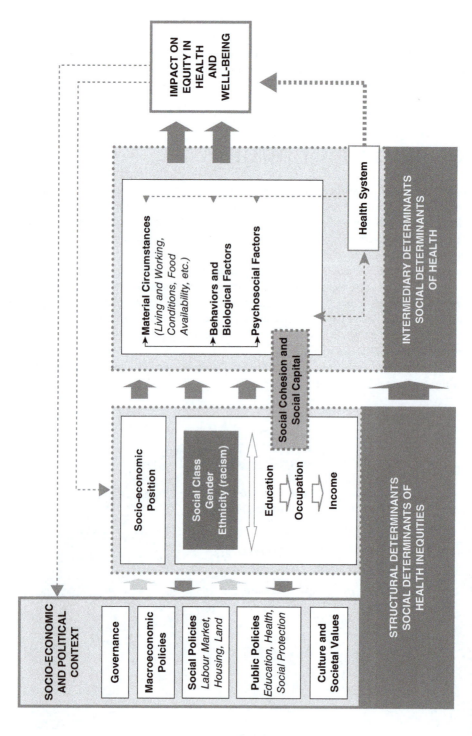

Figure 1.5   Structural and intermediary determinants © WHO

Social determinants of health are ultimately shaped by the distribution of money, power and resources at an international, national and local level. They have a profound influence on health inequities and avoidable health differences between different groups of people within countries and between countries. As you can see in Figure 1.4, the way in which the social determinants of health work involve complex interactions between them, and the WHO (2010) provides a useful framework to help us understand this in more depth.

As shown in Figure 1.5, there are two broad types of social determinants that can lead to health inequities: structural and intermediary determinants.

Structural determinants are categorized into sections, the first being the socio-economic and the political context. Within these sections are further subsections to consider:

1. *Governance: how society makes decisions about health*
2. *Macroeconomic policies: how the overall economic market operates on a large scale*
3. *Public policies: how education can support health and social protection*
4. *Culture and societal values: how these can shape or impact health outcomes.*

(WHO, 2010)

Structural determinants can lead to the unfair distribution of material and monetary resources that shape a person's *socio-economic position*. Position infers a person's place in society, which can affect their exposure, vulnerability and outcomes to conditions that have an impact on their health. Socio-economic position includes education, occupation income, gender, ethnicity and social class, and in turn affects the *intermediary determinants* of health's material circumstances. For example, an individual on a lower income may live in inadequate housing conditions, which may in turn impact their psychological health and relationships. One important thing to point out is that social cohesion and social capital can bridge the socio-economic and intermediary positions. During the Covid-19 pandemic, social cohesion encouraged communities to make sacrifices and cooperate with each other for the wider benefits of access to provision.

Access to healthcare

We should consider how health systems can influence how easy it is for people to access care. There are different approaches to how individuals access healthcare. For example, the UK follows the Beveridge model (the NHS) which is paid for by taxation and is free at the point of provision. The United States operates a health insurance system which requires its citizens to purchase insurance to access healthcare provision. Europe generally has a mixed approach called the Bismarck model, which is a social health insurance model, paid for by both the employee and government. There are critiques of all these systems, and none is perfect in terms of access to provision and waiting times. Interestingly, research by Edwards (2018) indicates that funding mechanisms have little direct impact of the quality of care.

Geophysical location can impact access to healthcare. Some areas have access issues when centres of excellence or specialisms are located in cities which may be many miles away from a small, countryside village. Some centres, like Great Ormond Street Children's Hospital (GOSH), acknowledge this by providing parents with accommodation. Many others, however, do not.

Intermediary determinants influence health and health inequities. The links between these determinants are not linear; they are complex and can work in both directions. We know that low income and poor education can impact health. Equally, poor health can impact the ability to go to work, which leads to a lower income.

If a population is affected by high levels of disease, it can have a wider effect on socio-economic and political contexts. An example of this is Covid-19, which has devastated communities across the globe, both from a health and economic perspective.

During the early days of the Covid-19 pandemic in the UK (February–March 2020), great efforts were made to house street homeless (rough sleepers), as they were classed as vulnerable. Homeless hostel users were also rehomed to reduce the spread of infection, and infection control in homeless settings was closely monitored. However, in subsequent waves, provision became patchy as the national government cancelled the 'Everyone in' strategy. Examine Activity 1.2 and consider the young man's social determinants of health. What factors might have led to him being homeless?

Activity 1.2   Critical thinking

A young man attends the local A&E department. He appears unkempt and disorientated. You are working with the triage nurse. Prior to the patient coming into the room, the nurse tells you he is a regular attender to the department and that he just likes to visit for company.

The man reveals to you that he is homeless and has no family or friends he can go to for help. You notice there is blood on the sleeve of his lower arm. You take him into the minor injuries unit and begin his initial assessment.

- What social determinants could be factors in this situation?
- What is available in your service to support your patient?

An outline answer is given at the end of the chapter.

People become homeless for many different reasons. The structural and intermediary causes would include social and socio-economic reasons, such as poverty, a lack of affordable housing, unemployment and insecure employment (the so-called gig economy). Life events also play an important role, such as family breakdown, poor mental health, substance misuse, leaving care, leaving prison and being an army veteran with no home to return to.

A closer look at the models

Pender's model

In 1982 (revised in 1996) Nola Pender created a health promotion model (HPM) to compliment traditional models of health promotion. The aim of her model is to support nurses and nursing associates in understanding the major determinants of health behaviours as a basis to promote healthy lifestyles. Pender noted that health professionals only intervened when an individual was already unwell, so her model focuses on motivation, positivity and prior life experiences. Pender et al. (2011) state that 'Health is positive, comprehensive, unifying, and humanistic. Health includes a disease component but does not make disease its principal element' (p. 4). The theory covers the life span for optimal health. Pender believed that by identifying wellness factors, and by influencing health behaviours, people and healthcare systems could save money.

People are the sum of their experiences, which then influence future choices. The social interactions that people have, and the competing demands they face, lead to behavioural outcomes. If you reflect back to Activity 1.1 and lay beliefs, you can see how Pender's model, outlined in more detail below, unites lay belief thinking with the social determinants of health.

Seven assumptions of Pender's model (2011)

1. People are motivated to affect conditions so they can achieve their human potential.
2. People can assess their competencies: they are self-aware.
3. People seek value in personal growth, they seek balance between stability and change.
4. People are active in regulating their actions.
5. People effect and are affected by their environment.
6. People are influenced by healthcare professionals.
7. Self-motivation is key to success.

Thirteen theoretical statements

1. Prior behaviour and characteristics influence belief and behaviours.
2. Benefits are instrumental in behaviour change.
3. Barriers play an important role in behaviour change.
4. Self-efficacy and competence increase the likelihood of behaviour change.
5. Self-efficacy reduces barriers to health behaviour.
6. Positive affect towards behaviour increases self-efficacy.
7. Increased commitment and action result from positive emotions and affect.
8. Significant others are influential in behaviour.
9. Interpersonal influences impact health promoting behaviour.
10. Situational influences impact health promoting behaviour.
11. The greater commitment to a plan of care the more likely the health promoting behaviour can be maintained over time.
12. Competing demands that require immediate attention will reduce the likelihood of engaging with the desired behaviour.
13. Cognition affect and environment can be modified to create incentives for health action.

The health belief model

In 1952, Hochbaum, Rosenstock, and Kegels contributed to the development of the health belief model (HBM) which suggests that an individual's willingness to change their health behaviors is primarily due to their perceptions of health. The model was developed after Hochbaum and colleagues noticed a significantly low response rate to tuberculosis screening. They believed that low uptake of the screening programme was driven by the two elements: firstly, an individual's motivation and secondly their perception of the illness. This combination produced what they refer to as a health belief. This theory is an early construct of the health belief model; however, the idea is still very much present in today's society.

The questions that Hochbaum et al. (1952) posed were:

- How will this disease affect me?
- How will a behaviour change benefit me?
- Do I have the skills necessary to change my own health behaviours?

Health behaviours are complex. We must ensure that any information we give is correct, and that it will meet the needs of the target audience. Demographic variables include children, young people, adults and older people, and must be inclusive of those with mental health issues and learning difficulties.

Hochbaum et al. refer to the six constructs that affect the thought process of the health belief model. These are explored in the box below in relation to problem drinking.

The six constructs applied to problem drinking:

1. *Perceived susceptibility*: The individual feels threatened or at risk enough for the behaviour to change. For instance, the danger resulting from alcoholism. There were almost 1.3 million alcohol-related hospital admissions in the UK in 2020.

2. *Perceived severity*: The individual develops an understanding that engaging in these unhealthy behaviours will be severe and that urgent action to change their behaviour is necessary. For instance, the knowledge that chronic alcoholism leads to death. In 2018, there were 7,551 alcohol-specific deaths. This is the second-highest level since the records began in 2001 (NHS, 2020).

3. *Perceived benefits*: The belief that positive outcomes can occur by changing behaviour. For example, by reducing alcohol dependence, the individual increases their life expectancy.

4. *Perceived barriers*: The actual or manifested cost, this can be monetary or material. Reminding the individual of the huge costs to their wealth and health will help to motivate and maintain the behaviour change.

5. *Cues to action*: These are external events that motivate the individual to want to change. The goal is to support people in their belief they can make the change. Individuals are supported to take responsibility for their own choices. This might be prompting them to consider the impact drinking has on a cherished relationship.

6. *Self-efficacy*: This is about the individual having the confidence to change. By taking small manageable steps and setting goals that are realistic to achieve.

You should note that this is an individual, personal health maintenance theory, and so not applicable to social or environmental issues. There will be some disparity between populations and individuals as not as everyone has the same access to health services, education or income. Using just one approach for one group or individual will not always lead to a successful outcome.

We will now discuss Tannahill and Beattie's models and compare all the models with Naidoo and Wills typology.

Tannahill's model

Tannahill (1985) defined health promotion as three overlapping spheres, which includes prevention, health education and health protection. A relatively simple idea, this model lays the foundations of the fundamental principles of health promotion but does not consider an individual's wellbeing.

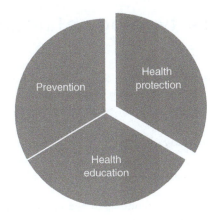

Figure 1.6 Tannahill's model

Beattie's model

Beattie's (1991) model looks at health promotion from two different approaches.

One axis looks at the level of intervention that individuals, population or communities require. The other axis looks at the approach taken to health promotion. If you examine Figure 1.7, you can see that at one end the approach is authoritative, while the other end is negotiated.

Combining the axis together creates four quadrants. These are health persuasion, legislative action, community development and personal counselling. Beattie argues these are the components that make up health promotion. An example of this is the national smoking ban. This is a policy which has a top-down approach. However, it is aimed at the collective population. Smoking cessation clinics, on the other hand, are negotiated and mediated by the individual via the counselling approach.

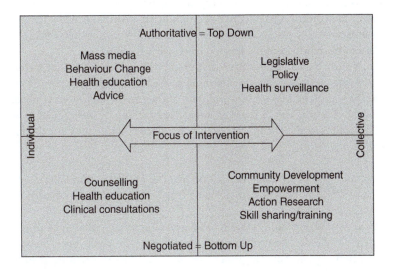

Figure 1.7 Beattie's model

Naidoo and Wills' typology of health promotion

Naidoo and Wills (2000) developed a typology of health promotion. Their typology is derived from components of previous research and identifies elements of similarity. Naidoo and Wills argued that health promotion has five different elements to it:

1. *Medical*: A medical preventative approach (for instance annual health checkups for individuals at risk);
2. *Education*: Providing people with information to make informed choices about their health;
3. *Behaviour change*: Encouraging individuals to change their attitudes towards their own health and in turn adopt healthier behaviours;
4. *Empowerment approach*: Offering support to develop a sense of self belief and self-efficacy;
5. *Social change approach*: Using research to influence policy (local and national) regarding accessible resources for health and social care.

Activity 1.3   Reflection

Look back over the models of health promotion and make notes of the main principles. Are all of these principles covered by Naidoo and Wills' typology? What other principles or elements of health promotion would you include if you were writing your own typology?

As this activity is based on your own ideas, there is no model answer provided.

Health promotion and children

So far, we have looked at health promotion theory and models. Now let us think about children and young people and where health behaviours begin. Children are influenced by their environment and the people who care for them. Health promotion principles are applied within the early years and health behaviours are intrinsically formed when we are young.

Bandura et al.'s work on social cognitive theory (1961) emphasised the importance of social learning. His work strongly denotes that learning and cognitive development relies on social influence. Bandura indicates that an integral part of human development is observation and the influence of those around us. If these elements are lacking or missing, people are unable to develop the appropriate social cognitive skills. Bandura categorises the principles of social cognitive theory:

1. *Observational learning*: By socialising, this teaches children many different behaviours through observation, observational learning is a key component of behavioural psychology.
2. *Modelling and imitation:* This refers to children observing the actions of others around them, in turn they learn how to behave. Modelling was discovered during Bandura's research. It demonstrated how children observe and imitate the actions of adults.
3. *Shaping:* The process of modifying a child's behaviour. This process is accomplished through instructing a child how to behave and rewarding them when they have succeeded. This was influenced by B.F. Skinner's notions of operant conditioning.

In his research, Bandura separates observational learning into four stages. These stages reflect the process of observing a behaviour in someone else and adopting the observed behaviour.

The four stages of observational learning

1. *Attention*: To learn a behaviour through social learning, the behaviour must first grab a child's attention. For the behaviour to attract a child's attention, it must be attractive to them in some way. Attraction then leads to attention. Sometimes children are drawn to the consequence of the behaviour they are seeing.
2. *Retention*: When a child's attention has been captured, they may retain what they saw. By retention, this can mean whether the observer will remember what they observed. The more the person remembers the behaviour, the more likely they are to imitate it.
3. *Reproduction*: When the observer has watched and remembered a model for behaviour. If the observer appreciated the behaviour, they may try to recreate it. An observer will hold the skills needed to reproduce the observed behaviour.
4. *Motivation*: This is the final stage of observational learning. Motivation is a crucial component in observational learning. For a behaviour to be reproduced regularly, there must be incentive for the behaviour.

Bandura's work on how we learn behaviours has important implications for health promotion. Indeed, his social cognitive theory shifts the field of health from a disease-based model to a health-based model that focuses on strategies for disease prevention and health promotion that enable healthier behaviour (Bandura, 1998).

To recap so far, we have looked at the different health promotion models and approaches, the theory of learned behaviour and how health promotion strategies can enable healthier lifestyles. We have already established that the most appropriate health promotion approach will depend on both the individual and the distinct circumstances you are working in; one size does not fit all.

Health promotion and mental health

We have looked at the application of health promotion models in relation to lifestyle changes. What if your patient engages in health behaviours that have developed due to a mental health condition but which are now impacting their physical health?

For instance, an eating disorder, such as anorexia or bulimia, is a mental health condition that can have significant implications for one's physical health. How can the health promotion models considered in this chapter be applied in practice to support a patient with an eating disorder?

Anorexia and bulimia are serious mental health conditions which have many similarities in origin. Men and women of any age can develop anorexia, but it is more common to develop in young women and typically starts in the mid-teens (NHS, 2020).

Walsh (2013) recognises that adolescence is a turbulent time, and his research has shown that individuals are most sensitive to the idea of reward during this time in their lives. Greenfield (2014) makes an interesting point in relation to social learning theory and the way in which it connects to anorexia. The media portrays images of excessively skinny women and men as positive. For developing adolescents, this sends a message that skinny is the dominant cultural image and some will go to extreme lengths to emulate that image.

Linking this to Bandura's social cognitive theory and learned behaviours in children, this has the potential to continue into adolescence. Walsh suggests that this increased sensitivity and rewarding element may contribute to, and explain why, adolescents are susceptible to developing eating disorders.

Walsh describes positive and negative reinforcements combined with increased sensitivity to rewarding actions. He outlines a number of reasons which may indicate what he describes as restricting patterns towards eating, which in turn can lead to a deep-seated unhealthy relationship with food. Walsh (2013) identifies these reasons below:

1. *Persistent and repeated dieting*: This leads to overtrained and highly practiced entrenched behaviour.
2. *Intermittent rewards*: These provide a strong reinforcement and the positive effects of the individual feeling they have accomplished something. By eating less (achieving a goal) *and* the effects of numbing emotions are much more reinforcing.
3. *Onset of anorexia nervosa*: This usually coincides with stress and some individuals learn better when they are stressed. So, behaviours that are acquired during a time of stress are more likely to become habits than when they are learned at other times.
4. *Weight loss*: This can lead to compulsive, obsessive and rigid patterns of thought and behaviour. The most cited example of this is the 'Minnesota starvation study' (1945), where healthy subjects developed symptoms of obsessionality much like anorexia nervosa patients following a period of starvation.

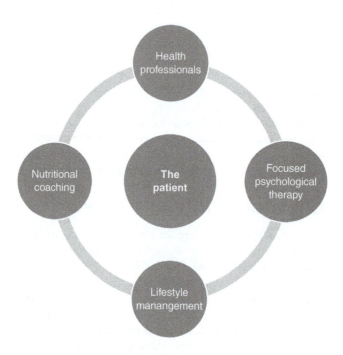

Figure 1.8   Cycle of intervention

When we feel stress, we need to release that stress. The mind, therefore, will naturally take us back to similar situations when we dealt with stress. Stress affects many of us for an array of reasons, for instance, due to relationships, school or work. For individuals who suffer from an eating disorder, additional factors such as environmental and social aspects may increase stress levels, causing harmful mental and behavioural patterns. Bennett and Murphy (1998) explain that stress is not a singular concept. It is a process that involves complex connections between the environment, physiological and psychological processes. Establishing the relationship between stress and health can allow individuals to define stressors for themselves, for them to truly address stressful triggers.

It is important that your patients are supported to understand the relationship between their stressful experiences and poor eating habits. Elements of intensive adolescent focused psychotherapy includes health promoting educational interventions. This includes supporting the patient to understand what they need to do to be healthy and teaching an understanding of the physiological effects of under or over-eating. You can draw on the health promotion models we have covered to do this, such as Pender's model and Naidoo and Wills' typology. Gleissner (2017) states that 'Engaging in habitual patterns can develop into a coping mechanism'. Aspects of Pender's model refer to self-efficacy beliefs supporting individuals to develop the confidence to change by taking small manageable steps, and by setting goals that are realistic to achieve for healthier lifestyle choices.

Coping mechanisms

Researchers such as Ekern (2016) and Chowdary (2020) have defined three kinds of coping: problem-focused, emotion-focused and perception-focused coping. Depending on the situation, the individual will differ as to how they will respond:

1. *Problem-focused coping: The individual will take direct action on their surroundings or themselves to remove or attempt to change the threat.*
2. *Emotion-focused coping: When the individual uses actions or thoughts to control unpleasant feelings brought on by the threat.*
3. *Perception focused coping: Cognitive attempts to reduce or alter the severity of a threat.*

(Ekern, 2016)

Chowdary (2020) states that 'In psychology, coping skills or coping strategies are a set of adaptive tools that we proactively administer to avoid burnout. These tools can be our thoughts, emotions, and actions and are dependent on our personality patterns' (p. 1).

There is increasing evidence to suggest that due to mental health issues, such as depression and anxiety, individuals engage in unhelpful behaviours. Holland (2019) states that

alcohol use disorder and depression are two conditions that often occur together. What is more, one can make the other worse in a cycle that is pervasive and problematic if not addressed and treated. Alcohol use can cause or worsen symptoms of mood disorders. Depression may even cause people to begin consuming large amounts of alcohol.

The WHO have a clear vision for mental health promotion 'Mental health is an integral part of health; indeed, there is no health without mental health' (WHO, 2018).

Mental health promotion encompasses actions that aim to improve wellbeing from a psychological perspective. The WHO indicates a variety of ways to promote mental health:

- early childhood interventions and support to children;
- socio-economic empowerment of women;
- social support for elderly populations;
- programmes targeted at vulnerable people;
- mental health promotional activities in schools;
- mental health interventions at work;
- housing policies;
- violence prevention programmes;
- anti-discrimination laws and campaigns.

Mental health promotion is a fundamental aspect of health promotion and links with the wider agenda of public health and the socio-economic agenda. 'Mental health promotion should be mainstreamed into governmental and nongovernmental policies and programmes. In addition to the health sector, it is essential to involve the education, labour, justice, transport, environment, housing, and welfare sectors' (WHO, 2020a).

Older people and health promotion

As the population grows older and people live for longer, preventative health education programmes are key to keeping the older population healthy.

The WHO has stated that health promotion is for the entire population. However, there is increasing evidence to suggest that health promotion is not always as inclusive as it could be in relation to the older population.

Age is a protected characteristic under the Equality Act (2010) and thus health promotion polices should be inclusive. However, Golinowska (2016) stated that the elderly have long been neglected as the addressee of health promotion activities. The need to promote health among older people was first highlighted in the 1990s, before which it was commonly assumed that older generations were not a good target for health promotion as it was thought to be too late to change their lifestyle. Requiring the elderly to radically change their diet and start exercising was perceived as disturbing to their peace and wellness and thus a waste of resources that would not improve the quality of people's lives.

Research undertaken by Strumpel and Billings (2006) indicated that exercising, smoking cessation, limiting alcohol consumption, participating in learning activities and integrating in the community can help to prevent the development of many diseases. Cognitive activities are shown to inhibit the loss of functional capacity and ultimately improve quality of life and extend life expectancy. It is important to highlight that the engagement of health promotion activities in this study was among people under the age of 85. Health promotion for those aged over 85 was focused on ensuring that they had appropriate medical attention and that their carers were offered support, rather than making changes to their health behaviours.

Health promoting strategies for older people have three aims:

1. maintain and increase functional capacity;
2. maintain or improve self-care;
3. improve social experiences.

The thinking behind these aims contributes to and promotes independence of the elderly and aims to improve quality of life for individuals.

Working with older people requires sensitive and tactful communication skills. The WHO (2020a) suggests adopting the following points for more effective health promotion activities.

- *Make messages more relevant to older people. Tailored messages (for example, about the importance of physical activity in later years) can make the message appear more relevant and appealing.*
- *Target messages at specific groups of older people, such as gendered screening sessions. Matching information to an individual's characteristics can influence how older people think and feel about a health issue.*
- *Manage emotional distress. Emotional distress can be both a catalyst for and a saboteur of change; hence, it needs to be managed successfully to encourage behavioural change and maintenance of that change.*
- *Consider an older person's social support. As people age, their social networks decrease in size and networks may be more effective at promoting stability than change.*

The NHS Long Term Plan (LTP) (2019a) aims to relieve the pressure on services across England, so the first priority of the many areas identified is prevention.

Each element of the long-term plan has prevention at its heart, emphasizing an effort to move away from a system that simply treats, into one that also helps to keep people well for longer. The LTP recognizes good health is about more than healthcare alone, and that to be implemented effectively the NHS must work in partnership with local government.

(NHS, 2019a)

In many respects, physical and mental health are one entity, one in turn affects the other. 'Making every contact count' (MECC) is an approach to behavioural change that utilises the millions of day-to-day interactions that organisations and individuals have with other people to support them in making positive changes to their physical and mental health and wellbeing (HEE, 2016). Look at Activity 1.4, how could you use MECC to support Mrs Kowalski during her health review?

Activity 1.4   Evidence-based practice

You are on placement in a GP surgery, and you are asked to support the practice nurse with her chronic disease review patients. You meet Mrs Kowalski who has come to have her blood pressure review.

You begin the review and approach the question of how often Mrs Kowalski exercises. She tells you that prior to her being diagnosed with high blood pressure she enjoyed walking, and although her walks were not particularly long in duration, she felt better for getting out in the fresh air.

Mrs Kowalski tells you that she is worried that if she walks her blood pressure will go up. She then tells you she has not gone for a walk for the last three months.

1. Why do you think she feels this way?
2. What could you do to change Mrs Kowalski's way of thinking?
3. Which health promotion models could you use to guide your thinking?

Compare your answer with the model answer at the end of the chapter.

Screening programmes

As we have established, there are many health promotion models, theories and educational programmes. However, screening programmes support health promotion from a proactive and preventative standpoint. This reflects Naidoo and Wills' typology of integrating medical preventative measures into health promotion. The example given in Activity 1.4 around Mrs Kowalski's blood pressure review is an integration of medical prevention and the opportunity to engage with MECC to promote not just physiological health but mental health also.

Health education interventions are expected to enhance screening, and early detection and in turn reducing mortality and morbidity rates. The Office for National Statistics (2020) reported on avoidable mortality and identified deaths from causes which could have been avoided through timely and effective healthcare and public health interventions.

NHS screening programmes proactively approach millions of individuals offering individual testing for one of a range of serious diseases. Screening is medically proactive and is different from other health promotion activities. An example is the *Promotion of the Cervical Screening Programme,* which raises women's awareness of cervical cancer prevention and encourages women to have regular cervical cancer screening through various health promotion activities and in collaboration with other partners (NHS, 2020).

Statistics

1. *Since the early 1970s, cervical cancer mortality rates have decreased by three-quarters (75 per cent) in females in the UK.*
2. *Over the last decade, cervical cancer mortality rates have decreased by around a fifth (21 per cent) in females in the UK.*
3. *Cervical cancer deaths in England are more common in females living in the most deprived areas.*

(Cancer Research, 2020)

There are many screening programmes in the UK. Following the appropriate training and competency-based assessment, you may undertake cervical smears when working within general practice settings.

Enhancing the skill base of registered nursing associates, with the appropriate competency-based training in cervical screening, will:

1. *Increase the number of sample takers across the country.*
2. *Improve access to screening.*
3. *Support screening's aim to reduce the incidence of cervical cancer and reduce the number of women who die from it.*

(PHE, 2019)

As a nursing associate, you will play an especially important role in engaging and encouraging women to attend their test as well as undertaking the procedure. Research has indicated that there are a number of barriers that prevent women from attending appointments, including embarrassment and worrying about the outcome of the test.

There is a clear link here with Hochbaum et al. and the six constructs within the health belief model on page 15. Improving knowledge and educating women about the benefits of attending testing is vital to the prevention and detection of cervical cancer. It is estimated by UK researchers that in England, cervical screening currently prevents 70 per cent of cervical cancer deaths. However, if everyone attended screening regularly, 83 per cent could be prevented (Cancer Research, 2020).

Chapter summary

This chapter has examined the core principles of health promotion and shown they are dependent on the individual's needs and situation. We have discussed and examined the various theories and models and examined Naidoo and Wills' typology, which synthesises many elements of these models. You have also been encouraged to reflect on which elements of the models are most useful to you in your setting. This chapter has examined issues that are relevant across the life span, and the intrinsic links of physical health and mental health within individuals and groups. Through engagement with the activities included in this chapter, you can reflect on and develop your own practice.

Activities: brief outline answers

Activity 1.2 Critical thinking (page 14)

Homelessness is associated with enormous health inequalities, including lower life expectancy, higher morbidity and greater usage of acute hospital services. Homelessness is a key driver of poor health, but homelessness itself results from accumulated adverse social and economic conditions. Addressing this man's housing needs would reduce his reliance on the NHS and reduce costs to the health service. Very few NHS trusts have pathways for homeless people, and it is likely he will represent with street acquired injuries.

Activity 1.4 Evidence-based practice (page 23)

Hypertension (high blood pressure) is the second biggest known global risk factor for disease, after poor diet. In the UK, high blood pressure is the third biggest risk factor for disease after tobacco smoking and poor diet. Around a third of adults in the UK have high blood pressure and it usually does not present with symptoms. All adults over the age of 40 are advised to get their blood pressure checked every five years. Addressing Mrs Kowalski's way of thinking, offering reassurance, combined with regular blood pressure monitoring and health education, would increase her level of exercise and reduce her blood pressure levels. MECC could be talking about her enjoyment of walking and how much it makes her feel better to get out in the fresh air.

Further reading

In order to understand the concept of the social determinants of health and how health is predicated on life chances, read Dahlgren, G. and Whitehead, M. (1991) *Polices and Strategies to Promote Social Equity in Health* found at www.euro.who.int/__data/assets/pdf_file/0010/74737/E89383.pdf

To familiarise yourself with the work of Albert Bandura and social cognitive theory, you might start with Bandura, A. (1998) 'Health promotion from the perspective of social cognitive theory', as it will introduce you to the concepts in an accessible format. This can be found at www.uky.edu/~eushe2/Bandura/Bandura1998PH.pdf

It would be helpful for you to read the NHS long term plan, so you get an understanding of the aims and goals behind many of the health promotion interventions discussed in this chapter. This can be found at www.longtermplan.nhs.uk/

Useful websites

Below are websites that will help in your research. They include NHS and WHO sites for information about different populations. Also included are websites for PHE and NHS health promotion campaigns. Always ensure that you get your information from academically acceptable sites and use original sources where possible.

Resources for information on global and UK populations:

Community profiles: fingertips.phe.org.uk/profile/health-profiles

National statistics: www.nomisweb.co.uk/

The World Health Organization, coronavirus: www.who.int/health-topics/coronavirus#tab=tab_1

Public Health England: www.gov.uk/government/organisations/public-health-england

NHS health promotion resources:

Anorexia nervosa – Treatment – NHS: www.nhs.uk

Change4Life: www.nhs.uk/change4life

Change for Life Evidence Review: assets.publishing.service.gov.uk/government/uploads/system/uploads/attachment_data/file/774106/Change4Life_Evidence_review_26062015.pdf

Exercise as you get older: www.nhs.uk/live-well/exercise/exercise-as-you-get-older/

MECC fact sheet: www.makingeverycontactcount.co.uk/media/27613/mecc-resources-fact-sheet-v9-20180601.pdf

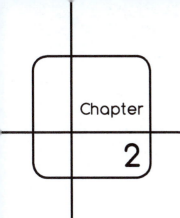

Chapter 2

Communication skills in health promotion

Ami Jackson

> # Chapter aims
>
> After reading this chapter, you will be able to:
>
> 1. understand how anatomy and physiology and cognition work together for communication;
> 2. understand how to develop your interpersonal skills;
> 3. determine how to act as a behaviour change agent using communication skills;
> 4. examine case studies written by nursing associates to improve your practice.

Introduction

In March 2020, the poet Michael Rosen became seriously ill with coronavirus. He was put into an induced coma, and at the end of his bed his nurses kept a diary for him. His nurses wrote notes and messages of good will and hope, hope that he would recover and read them. Rosen had written a poem called 'These are the hands' prior to becoming unwell. Someone typed it out and hung it above his bed. If you get a moment, read it, it was written for you. Poems are a form of communication that can indicate feelings, fears and longings, and the universality of love.

This chapter will introduce you to the science behind communication and theoretical models of communication. It will cover methods of communication to successfully deliver health promotion to patients and service users across all healthcare settings. This chapter will also incorporate the voice of nursing associates and their 'Lived experience' and will offer scenarios and activities to enhance your own development.

Communication is an art and a skill in itself. There are many intrinsic components to communication, it is something we do on a daily basis without really contemplating the process. As Peter Drucker's (1989) wise words indicate, the most important thing in communication is hearing what is not said. Communication is defined as 'the imparting, conveying, or exchange of ideas, knowledge and information'. This can apply to words or body language (Oxford Dictionary, 2020). Sibiya (2018) describes communication as a core component of sound relationships, collaboration and cooperation, which in turn are essential aspects of professional practice. Sibiya (2018) argues that the quality of the communication and interactions delivered by nursing associates has a major influence on patient outcomes and reduces errors. As a nursing associate if you use effective communication and interpersonal skills, you can enhance your professional practice.

Burnard and Gill (2008) points out that we have a common tendency to think that communication is focused just on speech, conversation or written documents. When, in fact, communication itself is much more. For example, we communicate through the clothes we wear, our hair styles, the jewellery we wear and religious symbols we adopt, and by doing so we are conveying a message about who we are.

The NMC's *Professional Standards of Practice and Behaviour for Nurses, Midwives and Nurse Associates* (2018) otherwise known as 'The Code' states you must communicate clearly and apply the following:

1. *Use terms that people in your care, colleagues and the public can understand.*
2. *Take reasonable steps to meet people's language and communication needs, providing, wherever possible, assistance to those who need help to communicate their own or other people's needs.*

3. Use a range of verbal and nonverbal communication methods, and consider cultural sensitivities, to better understand and respond to people's personal and health needs.
4. Check people's understanding from time to time to keep misunderstanding or mistakes to a minimum.
5. Be able to communicate clearly and effectively in English.

Let's examine the science

We must consider how we communicate with our patients, staff and relatives every day. Communication is a vast topic depending on which way you choose to look at it, so let us start with the science. The human brain is believed to function in a complex chemical environment through various types of neurons and neurotransmitters. Neurons are brain cells and we have billions, they are capable of instant communication with each other through chemical messengers called neurotransmitters (Ankrom, 2019). There are tiny hair cells in our inner ear, these send electrical signals to the auditory nerve. This is connected to the auditory centre of the brain, and where the electrical impulses are perceived by the brain as sound. The brain translates the impulses into sounds that we know and understand. Hearing is a biomechanical activity, but understanding is a cognitive activity. Examine the flow chart in Figure 2.1 to see how hearing happens within the ear and how it reaches the brain.

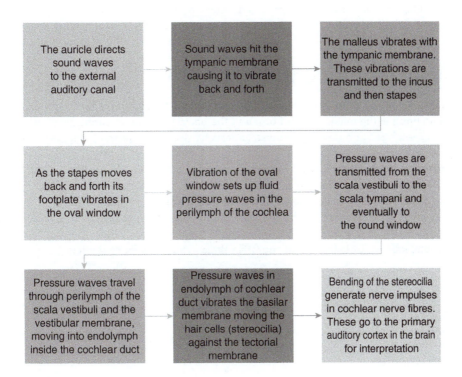

Figure 2.1   How hearing happens © SAGE

The neuron

Examine Figure 2.2, you can see that the middle of the neuron is referred to as the cell *body or soma*. Inside the nucleus is the cell's genetic material (DNA). This determines what type of cell it is and how it will work. The *dendrites are situated at the end of the cell body* and receives information which is transmitted from other neurons. The *axon terminal is situated at the other end of the cell body*; it is a long tubular shape that expands away from the cell body. The axon conducts electrical signals away from the cell, the axon terminal also holds vesicles where neurotransmitters are stored. The *nodes of Ranvier* are the small cavities between the myelin insulation of Schwann cells which line the axon. The main function of myelin is to *protect and insulate these axons and enhance (speed up) the electrical conduction*.

Neurotransmitters

The brain cells receive sensory information as electrical impulses which travel down the axon to the axon terminal where neurotransmitters are stored. This initiates a release of transmitters into the synapse, a small space between the delivering neuron and the obtaining (receiving) neuron. As you can see from Figure 2.3, the neurotransmitter attaches to a receptor and the message travels along the next neuron in a lightning-fast transaction.

Speech

Speech is generated by the supra-laryngeal vocal tract (SVT) to produce the voice and begins in the diaphragm. Air comes from the lungs and passes through the vocal folds. The tongue makes the shape of sounds and the upper and lower lips, upper and lower teeth, and the roof of our mouth (alveolar ridge, palate, velum) and nose in order to make specific sounds and words (see Figure 2.4).

Communication and the brain

As we have mentioned, there are billions of neurons that are situated inside the human brain. The human brain is the most powerful organ in the body. Waugh and Grant (2018) define the brain as 'the enlarged and developed mass of nervous tissue that forms the upper end of the central nervous system'.

The brain is divided into four lobes frontal, parietal, temporal and occipital. Each lobe is responsible for controlling what we see, taste, smell, hear and touch. The cerebellum receives messages from other sensory systems and it also regulates movement. Each lobe works in synchronisation with the other, for the purposes of this chapter, let us briefly look at the frontal lobe.

The frontal lobe controls important cognitive skills in humans, for example:

- emotional expression;
- problem solving;
- memory;
- language;
- judgement;
- sexual behaviour.

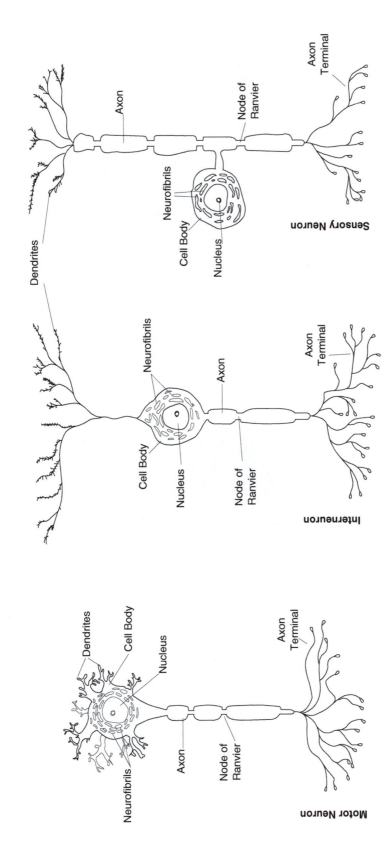

Figure 2.2   The neuron

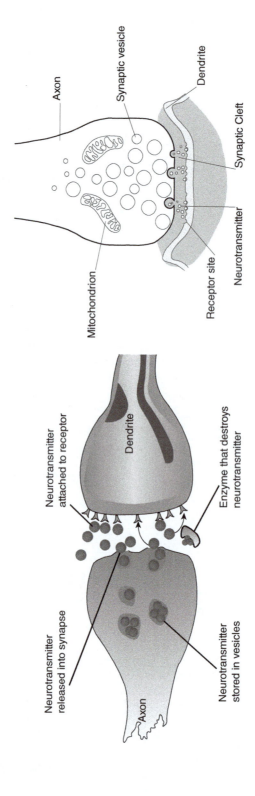

Figure 2.3 Neurotransmitters

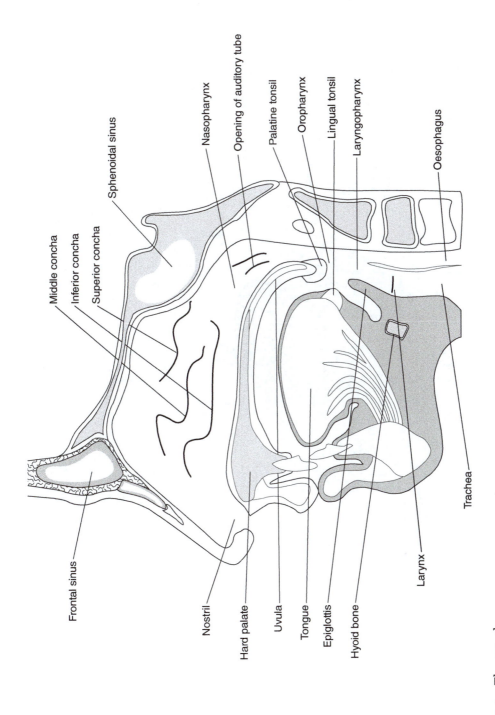

Frontal sinus

Middle concha
Inferior concha
Superior concha

Sphenoidal sinus

Nasopharynx

Opening of auditory tube

Palatine tonsil

Oropharynx

Lingual tonsil

Laryngopharynx

Oesophagus

Nostril

Hard palate

Uvula

Tongue

Epiglottis

Hyoid bone

Larynx

Trachea

Figure 2.4   The mouth

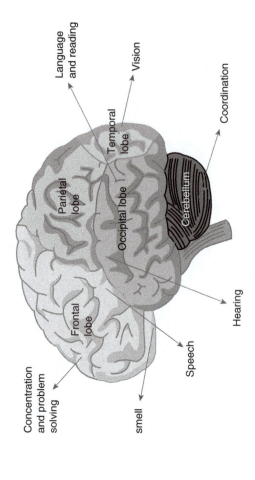

Figure 2.5 The brain

The frontal lobe *controls* our personalities and most importantly it enables us to communicate. Activity 2.1 now asks you to consolidate your learning from this first part of the chapter.

Activity 2.1   Critical thinking

Thinking about what you have learned so far, what physiological factors could prevent someone from hearing, speaking to and understanding you.

Write a list and compare with the list at the end of the chapter.

Having looked at the science behind communication, we now turn to studying communication models.

Communication models

There are several types of communication models such as Schramm (1954), Shannon and Weaver (cited in Ritch, 1986) and Berlo (1960). Berlo's (1960) sender, message, channel, receive (SMCR) model of communication is linear meaning the 'line' of communication is a one-way process, whereby the sender delivers a message to the receiver. The communication skills of the sender and receiver affect how well the message is communicated. If the sender has poor communication skills, the receiver may not get the right message. And if the receiver is not a good communicator, they might misinterpret the message.

Attitude between the message sender and receiver can influence how successful the message is, the tone and phrasing used all have an impact. As does where the sender and receiver stand within a hierarchy or group. The knowledge of the sender and receiver has an impact on understanding the message. The type of language used, acronyms, jargon and technical language can all act as barriers to the success of the message. Language, values, beliefs and life experiences can help or hinder deliverance and acceptance of a message. Consider the scepticism that resulted from the government's mixed messages regarding mask-wearing during the Covid-19 pandemic, the message should be clear and consistent.

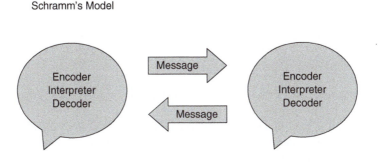

Figure 2.6   Schramm's model

Communication is a complex process. In fact, messages are sent simultaneously, and more than one message can be sent when communicating. We will discuss the effect of body language on communication further in this chapter. The channel chosen to communicate can impact on the effectiveness of the message. In nursing, this might be using handwritten notes versus using electronic notes, emails versus text messages, a phone call versus a message left on voice mail. You need to decide which is the most effective means of delivering a message.

An interactive communication model means 'a mutual or reciprocal action' and is a two-way process. Schramm's model (1954) builds upon linear theory. Both the sender and receiver encode and decode the message in order to understand it correctly.

The Shannon and Weaver transactional model is 'meaning relating to exchange or interaction between people'. This model is used for interpersonal communication, as it explains notions of simultaneous message sending, incorporating noise and feedback.

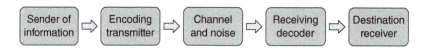

Figure 2.7 Shannon and Weaver's model

As you can see from the diagram, noise can interfere with the message, noise can be literally anything that prevents the message from being heard. It can be anything from a small distraction such a phone pinging, background chat, to intense pain.

Interpersonal skills

Interpersonal skills are the behaviours and strategies a person uses to interact with others effectively. You will interact daily with an array of clinical and medical personnel, patients, their families and other individuals. Your primary interpersonal skill is active listening, where you demonstrate to others that you are listening to and understanding their message. You can do that by verbally paraphrasing what they have said to ensure accuracy. You should maintain a calm and professional demeanour while communicating, as this inspires confidence. Examine Activity 2.2, how can James support the angry relative by using his interpersonal skills?

Much of our communication is done not with words but with our body. Body language is a nonverbal communication, and we tend to trust body language more than words. We will examine this further in the chapter.

Case study 2.1: James

James is a nurse associate on a busy surgical ward. It is visiting time and a patient's daughter is waiting to see him at the nurse's station.

James introduces himself and asks how he can help. The relative responds angrily. She looks stressed and is waving her arms. She shouts at James, saying that her mother has been left in a chair and is unable to reach her drink.

Her mother has dementia and suffers from re-occurring urinary tract infections (UTIs). The angry relative reiterates that she has told several staff members this and no one is listening to her. She insists she wants to speak to the ward manager.

Activity 2.2   Critical thinking

- What type of communication models could have been used here?
- Who could James speak to about the concerns raised?
- What skills might James have to use to initially deal with the situation?

Compare your answer to the answer at the end of the chapter.

Here are some useful facts that may be helpful when dealing with situations like the one James had to deal with. NHS England research focused on the root causes of patient dissatisfaction and found that poor communication lay at the heart.

1. Seventy per cent of Root Cause Analysis completed within the NHS noted that lack of clear communication was a contributing factor to poor patient experience (NHS England, 2015).
2. Ineffective communication among healthcare professionals is one of the leading causes of error and patient harm (NHS England, 2015).
3. Communication failures lead to increases in harm, length of stay and resource use, as well as reducing staff morale (NHS England, 2015).
4. Poor communication is one of the most common causes for dissatisfaction with health services. Research evidence shows the strong links between team communication and clinical outcomes (RCN, 2019a).

Body language

Body language is nonverbal communication and includes facial expressions, gestures, posture and tone of voice. These are powerful communication tools. When you are physically communicating with someone, you are continuously giving and receiving wordless signals. You should remember that few of us are good natural liars. If you are saying one thing, but your face and body are saying another, body language is more likely to be believed. Try to keep an open assured relaxed posture, maintain eye contact (without staring) and think about how you speak (pitch, tone, inflection), and non-word verbal sounds (such as 'um').

When talking to your patient, you read your patient's body language at the same time. Do their words match the body language? Is their face relaxed and at ease or is it tense? How are they holding their body, do they look in pain and in discomfort? Compare what they say with what you see.

Your facial expression can convey far more words than you speak. Facial expressions for emotions, such as happiness, sadness, anger, surprise and fear, are near universal across all cultures.

Culture and communication

Culture is often depicted as the mixture of a body of knowledge, a body of belief and a body of behaviour. It involves numerous components that are often specific to ethnic, racial, religious, geographic or social groups. This includes personal identification, language, thoughts, communications, actions, customs, beliefs, values and institutions. For the provider of health information or healthcare, these elements influence beliefs and belief systems surrounding health, healing, wellness, illness, disease and delivery of health services. The National Institute for Health (NIH, 2021) suggests the idea of cultural respect has an encouraging effect on patient care delivery, enabling providers to deliver services that are respectful of and responsive to the health beliefs, practices and cultural and linguistic needs of diverse patients. Culture is important, as it sends a message about who we are and who our patients are. We need to seek to understand and embrace cultural differences through clear communication.

Another important aspect to consider is body language and gestures. An example of this can be found in some Arab and African countries, where greeting the opposite sex by shaking hands or hugging is considered ill-mannered or even a moral crime. This is different to the western world, where it is a common practice to do this in order to appear welcoming (Akkilinc, 2019).

Values and beliefs are another aspect to consider in healthcare. For instance, some societies are very patriarchal, and the father or eldest son makes all the decisions for the family. Other cultures also have different ideas about modesty, and they will object to revealing examination gowns, preferring a robe.

Language is a barrier for those for whom English is not a first language. Patients do not always understand procedures or the need for them. They may not have a good understanding of the importance of taking medications (at set times, before or after food), and may not understand discharge information received from healthcare professionals. Therefore, it is essential these barriers are overcome to support health.

Methods of communication

Communication is something we do every day. It comes in a variety of formats verbal, nonverbal and written. It is not just the method that we use; it is also the interpersonal skills that come with communicating.

It is important to recognise that this is a skill you need to work at to develop. Think of your mind as a communication toolbox. In any given situation you will select a tool that is appropriate to the situation and enables you to interact with others in a positive way. You may use one or all of them at once, we call these interpersonal skills.

- As we discovered earlier, listening is the active process of receiving and responding to spoken (and sometimes unspoken) messages.
- Open-ended questions are a great way to get more information from the person answering your question. By their very nature, they beg for more details. Open-ended questions are questions which need thinking about and require more than a short, fixed response.
- Closed questions are questions to which you would typically receive a yes or no answer.

Examples might be:
Hello Mr Ajay, would you like a cup of tea? (closed)
Hello Mr Ajay, what would you like to drink? (open)
Hello Mr Ajay, have you had a cup of tea? (closed)
Hello Mr Ajay, when did you last have a drink? (open)

Communication methods are multifaceted and complex. Arguably, communication is interlinked into many other elements of care. We have discussed how we communicate through questioning, listening and observing. We will now look at record keeping and documentation.

Record keeping

Record keeping and documentation is a fundamental and legal practice that all professionals must follow. If it is not written down, it did not occur in the eyes of the law. Most importantly, it is a method of written or electronic communicative evidence. There are nine key principles that should always be applied:

1. *Records should be completed at the time, or as soon as possible after the event.*
2. *All records must be signed, timed and dated if handwritten. If digital, they must be traceable to the person who provided the care that is being documented.*

3. *Ensure that you are up to date in the use of electronic systems in your place of work, including security, confidentiality and appropriate usage.*
4. *Records must be completed accurately and without any falsification and provide information about the care given as well as arrangements for future and ongoing care.*
5. *Jargon and speculation should be avoided.*
6. *When possible, the person in your care should be involved in the record keeping and should be able to understand what the records say.*
7. *Records should be readable when photocopied or scanned.*
8. *In the rare case of needing to alter a record, the original entry must remain visible (draw a single line through the record) and the new entry must be signed, timed and dated.*
9. *Records must be stored securely and should only be destroyed following your local policy.*

(RCN, 2021)

Patient-centred care and communication

Patient-centred care and communication go hand in hand. No decision should be made without a patient's collaboration and informed consent. In order to do this, communication is vital. Kindness and respect mean different things to different people, which is why it matters in person-centred care. Being person-centred means thinking about what makes each person unique and doing everything you can to put their needs first (NMC, 2020). The National Institute for Clinical Excellence (NICE) support the NMC, stating that all patients should have the opportunity to make informed decisions about their care and treatment in partnership with their healthcare professionals. Exploring decision making and communication is also an important factor that is included in the communication process. The NHS Constitution for England states that 'services must reflect, be coordinated around, and tailored to the needs and preferences of patients' (Gov.UK, 2012, 2021) and that engaging people in their own care helps them to actively manage their health and wellbeing.

Communicating with people who have communication difficulties

You will care for patients who have little or no speech, little or no hearing or patients who are difficult to understand. They may have difficulty in forming or remembering words. They may also have difficulty in understanding you. Communication difficulties can occur alongside other diagnoses or form part of another disability. Some difficulties may be lifelong, such as deafness, or a learning disability, such as Down's syndrome or cerebral palsy. Some are acquired through a traumatic injury, or through developing a mental health disorder, such as schizophrenia or post-traumatic stress disorder (PTSD). Some occur as part of age-related ailments, such as dementia (howsoever caused) and hearing loss.

It can be challenging to communicate with people with a learning disability (LD), but essential that you do so. There is a danger of diagnostic overshadowing, this is where a behaviour is assumed to be part of the disability rather than an indication of pain or trauma. People with LD suffer poor health outcomes as either they are not diagnosed until too late or because of failed communication strategies. People with LD can exhibit challenging behaviours, and this often upsets both ward patients and the staff. In reality, people with LD are often scared in unfamiliar surroundings, and no one gives them the reassurance they need. Some people with LD suffer from social anxiety and social communication disorder (SCD), which can adversely impact their care. It is important that speech and language therapy services are included in any therapeutic care plan.

Good communication is needed not just with the patient with LD but with their care providers. This could be family or staff from a dedicated setting. It is helpful that the patient with LD has someone who can speak for them (an advocate), or someone who knows them well, and knows how to communicate with the patient in their preferred manner. The patient's medical notes should include details of their preferred communication method, such as cards with signs and symbols showing objects of reference the patient can point to, or Makaton sign language. You should give close attention to nonverbal expressions, such as body position, facial gestures and other nonverbal signs that may indicate pain or anxiety. If your patient with LD exhibits a behaviour such as rocking, hair pulling or tummy rubbing, check if this is normal, or if this is a behaviour which indicates discomfort.

Activity 2.3   Work-based learning

LD patients and their carers can download and print off a patient's passport to bring into hospital with them, you can find an example here: www.england.nhs.uk/6cs/wp-content/uploads/sites/25/2015/03/healthcare-passport.pdf

Look for other examples and study them to familiarise yourself with the information you need to communicate with your LD patient. Ask your supervisor if your placement uses passports and if they are kept with the patient's notes or at the bedside.

Communicating with deaf people requires patience. Ensure that the battery in their hearing aids, if they have them, is working, that the tube is not blocked by ear wax and that the aids are in the correct position in their ears. Speak slowly and clearly and ensure that background noise is kept to a minimum. Sit or stand where your patient can see your facial expressions and body language. If they need to remove their hearing aids for a treatment, arrange signals they will understand.

People with dementia need to be spoken to using short sentences and they will need time to assimilate what you have said, and to formulate a response. They still have capacity for choice making, so they should be given two options at a time, then you should check for understanding before moving on. It is helpful to sit next to the patient, give a gentle touch to reassure them. People with dementia sometimes substitute words, as the word they want is not accessible. They might know they have used the wrong words and get frustrated at their recall inability. People with dementia are easily discombobulated and may react in inappropriate ways such as shouting, agitation or retreating into a sullen silence.

Decision-making concepts and communication

Decision making is an integral part of patient care and encapsulates the information communicated between patient and professional. NICE (2021) refer to decision making as a guide for nursing associates to assess, assimilate, evaluate and/or discard components of information to make good judgements in clinical and non-clinical situations. Although these situations may be fraught with conflict at times, it empowers people to make decisions about the treatment and care that is right for them at that time.

This is important when we are communicating in relation to the decisions we are making with our patients, we must continue to ask ourselves is this the right approach. This is an inductive approach, and this concept is dynamic. It changes over time in different contexts throughout nursing.

Hamm (1988) considered the notion of the cognitive continuum or a systematic process within professionals. Hamm implies that decisions are reached by the analysis of a situation and, depending on the specifics of that situation, can be influenced by the nursing associate's experience. Which leads us to heuristics. Heuristics is an aspect of decision making. It is subjective and an individualised approach that reflects on a nursing associate's own experiences to simplify a choice that is complex in nature. Simon (1990) is noted for work in heuristics and claimed that professionals seek to minimise the amount of effort that is linked to the decision-making process. Johansson and O'Brien (2015) refer to this as the rule of thumb or a mental short cut. Over-reliance on this type of knowledge base can mean that using cognitive shortcuts when handling information may stray from the principles of competent decision making.

Empathetic listening

When you communicate with your patient, it is important to show empathetic listening skills. Have you ever heard the phrase put yourself in other people's shoes? By doing this, you are understanding and sharing another person's feelings, paying special attention to how they feel and why. Building this skill boosts our own emotional intelligence and helps us as practitioners respond in a positive way towards our patients. Empathy is a powerful communication skill that is often misunderstood and underutilised. Initially, empathy was referred to as 'bedside manner'. Now, however, authors and educators consider empathetic communication a teachable, learnable skill that has perceptible benefits for both the professional and the patient. Effective empathetic communication enhances therapeutic effectiveness of the clinician–patient relationship. Appropriate use of empathy as a communication tool facilitates the clinical interview, increases the efficiency of gathering information, and honours the patient (Harris, 2021).

Some people confuse empathy with sympathy. They are two completely different things entirely. Longley (2020) states:

Sympathy is a feeling and expression of concern for someone, often accompanied by a wish for them to be happier or better off such as 'Oh dear, I hope the chemo helps'. In general, sympathy implies a deeper, more personal, level of concern than pity, which is a simple expression of sorrow. However, unlike empathy, sympathy does not imply that one's feelings for another are based on shared experiences or emotions. It is about connecting with your patient on an emotional level.

For example, your patient is suffering from poorly controlled blood sugars. They are not compliant with their medication because they believe they do not need it. They think that diet control has worked in the past, so will work again.

By understanding your patient's thinking, you are letting the patient know that you see their perspective. You may not agree with their opinion, but you are establishing a relationship using empathy.

Price (2017) explains that the nurse–patient rapport is established at the first meeting or interaction, and it develops throughout the therapeutic relationship. Initially, nursing associates should establish trust with the patient through the questions they ask, however, as care progresses, you will be required to address other issues that may challenge the relationship you have.

Empathy does not mean that you should automatically try to fix a problem that someone has. Quite often, you cannot fix someone's problems, but you can offer an empathetic ear (Bennett and Rosner, 2019). There are three elements to consider in order to give your patients the opportunity to talk and express how they feel.

1. It is important to be genuine in your approach when you listen.
2. Secondly, be aware of verbal and nonverbal cues; for example, you ask your patient how they are feeling, and they tell you they are fine, but their nonverbal facial expressions do not match what they are telling you.

3.   Thirdly, summarise back to your patient the information they have told you. This shows you have not only listened, but understood the information.

Read Case Study 2.1, this is a personal report by Bethany about an event which occurred during her practice placement. Think about how Bethany applied theory to practice.

Case study 2.2: Bethany

Bethany is a nursing associate on a placement in a busy medical ward. She has been looking after Mrs Adebayo who was admitted for general malaise and loose stools. Mrs Adebayo has received intravenous fluids. Mrs Adebayo has a history of peripheral vascular disease and has had a previous left leg amputation, she also has early onset dementia. She has begun to work with the physiotherapy staff on transfers from bed to chair when Bethany finds Mrs Adebayo tearful following her therapy, and asks her why she is upset. Mrs Adebayo tells Bethany that the physiotherapy team have said that, when she returns home, she will have to use a hoist as her transfers are unsafe. Bethany asked Mrs Adebayo about her mobility prior to coming into the ward. Mrs Adebayo replied that she had a prosthetic lower limb and before she became unwell, she walked with the prosthetic and two walking sticks. She went on to say she tried to tell the physiotherapist this, but the physiotherapist said there was nothing written in the notes about this. Bethany placed her hand on Mrs Adebayo's shoulder and reassured her she understood her views and why she was upset.

Activity 2.4   Communication

How do you think Bethany should use communication to support Mrs Adebayo?

Compare your answer with Bethany's at the end of the chapter.

Ratna (2019) states if either the patient or professional does not understand the intent of the information expressed, communication cannot be effective. Therefore, it is vital that the professionals not only communicate clearly with the patient but also between one another. As you can see from Bethany's interaction, a communication breakdown had occurred between the hospital, the patient and the care facility.

Ratna conveys a good example of this, describing how the role of a doctor is very different from the role of (say) an occupational therapist. However, both must communicate clearly with each other to ensure that appropriate care recommendations are met. Ratna then infers that patient–system interactions are bidirectional or, put simply, a two-way functional process. We can relate this to Schram's model of communication. The patients we care for need to be able to express information about their health issues. Professionals must receive that information and effectively understand information in order to treat and manage issues appropriately. They also need to communicate effectively across teams and settings. By doing so, they would reduce the likely hood of health concerns such as Mrs Adebayo's.

Ratna summed up helpful points to consider in relation to health literacy improvement processes, and gave strategies for clear communication:

- Give a warm greeting.
- Maintain eye contact.
- Listen carefully.
- Be aware of the patient's body language as well as your own.
- Speak slowly and concretely in non-medical language.
- Use graphic boards and demonstrations when appropriate.
- Encourage patient participation and questions.
- Document the conversation and share concerns.

Think about communication and health promotion. It is important to think about the way in which we address our patients. Here are some questions to consider and apply in your day-to-day practice.

- What is the issue or issues?
- What does the patient need to do and why?
- Why should the patient comply with what is being suggested?
- What should the patient expect in terms of outcome (both pros and cons)?
- Are there any alternatives (including no treatment)?

After any interaction with the patients we care for, it is vital that you and any other professional ensures the patient understands the healthcare issues that have been discussed. This needs to be confirmed with the patient. If confirmation is lacking, there is no assurance that patients will be able to perform the potentially intricate treatments that the healthcare professional expects of them.

The teach-back method has proved to be simple but effective way to check, not only a patients' condition but also to ensure the patient understands the explanation and advice given to them during each interaction (RCN, 2019).

Dinh et al. (2016) offer evidence from a systematic review, which supports the use of the teach-back method in educating people with chronic disease to maximise their understanding of their ailment. Dinh et al. consider this promotes knowledge, adherence, self-efficacy and self-care skills. Any information should be provided in a format that a patient understands, in order to engage in self-management. An example of this could be medication reconciliation and easy-to-read drug labels, or help and guidance leaflets in a variety of formats.

Communication tools

There are many tools that are used in healthcare. Although not all will be appropriate in all settings, you can apply the principles to the care you deliver to your patients. Rabøl et al.'s (2011) research analysed 84 root cause analysis incidents over a two-year period, which included descriptions and characteristics of communication errors such as handover errors and errors during teamwork.

An example of a communication tool is Situation, Background, Assessment and Recommendation, otherwise known as SBAR. Widely used throughout most trusts in the UK, it is designed to support staff sharing concise, focused information. The Institute for Healthcare Improvement (IHI) (2021) states:

SBAR is an easy-to-remember, concrete mechanism useful for framing any conversation, especially critical ones, requiring a clinician's immediate attention and action. It allows for an easy and focused way to set expectations for what will be communicated and how between members of the team, which is essential for developing teamwork and fostering a culture of patient safety.

Communication can be defined as 'a two-way process of reaching mutual understanding, in which participants not only exchange information, but also create and share meaning' (NHS Improvement, 2021).

Situation: Identify yourself and site you are calling from. Identify the patient by name and the reason for your report. Describe your concerns.

Background: Give the patient's reason for admission. Explain significant medical history. You then inform the other person of the patient's background. Include admitting diagnosis, date of admission, prior procedures, current medications, allergies, pertinent laboratory results and other relevant diagnostic results.

Assessment: Vital signs, clinical impressions, concerns

Recommendations: Explain what you need. Be specific about your request and any time frames. Make suggestions and clarify expectations.

(RCN, 2019)

Case Study 2.2 considers how Angie developed communication skills to support her patients through a procedure that required the patient to keep their head and neck absolutely still. The patient was unable to speak but had to communicate their wishes during the procedure. This was a tricky situation that needed to be resolved before the procedure could take place.

Case study 2.3: Angie

Angie is a qualified nursing associate working in interventional radiology. Working with a registered nurse, she has been allocated to the look after a patient during a gastroscopy procedure, providing reassurance and support. Angie's role is to ensure the patient remains calm, still and informed during the procedure whilst monitoring vital observations.

Prior to the procedure, Angie discussed with the patient a safe way to communicate their wishes during the test. When Angie asked a question the patient agreed with, they would raise their right hand. Or they would raise their left hand if they wanted the procedure to stop. The patient was anxious about the procedure. Angie took time to explain what to expect prior to the test, during the test and when the procedure was coming to an end. They agreed that Angie would say, 'We are down to the last part of the test now, we have approximately 5 mins left, can you raise your right hand if you are ok, or your left hand if you are not'. The patient tolerated the procedure and had their anxiety eased by the approach that was taken by Angie.

Activity 2.5   Work-based learning

How would you approach the patient in this situation? What communication methods would you adopt?

Now read Angie's reflective account at the end of the chapter.

Using communication to promote health

Health communication strategies aim to change people's knowledge, attitudes and behaviours. This can be done using mass media (TV, radio, print media), social media and small local (targeted, focused) campaigns. Local campaigns should be mindful of community make-up and ensure priorities for different cultures. Also, health literacy and internet access should be considered when attempting to target hard-to-reach groups. Effective health communication strategies are evidence-based using health promotion theories and models (see Chapter 1). Becker's (1974) health belief model was utilised. It states that two factors influence the adoption of a health protective behaviour:

1. a feeling of being personally threatened by a disease;
2. a belief that the benefits of adopting the protective health behaviour would outweigh the perceived costs of adopting that behaviour.

For instance, Covid-19 campaigns included national and local newspaper articles, television broadcasts and radio commercials, alongside public service announcements, newsletters, pamphlets, videos and many digital tools. The messages utilised three-word slogans as an effective concept carrier to raise awareness to:

1. increase risk perception of catching and transmitting Covid-19;
2. reinforce positive behaviours such as washing hands, wearing a mask, staying at home;
3. influence social norms such as not visiting other homes, shopping only when needed, testing and self-isolating;
4. increase availability of support services such as Nightingale hospitals, mass screening centres and mass vaccination centres.

And, despite bizarre and ill-founded conspiracy theories, many people adopted the health promotion messages to support and protect their own and their family's health.

National campaigns usually recruit a personality (or personalities) who are interested in the topic and who can appeal to their fan base. Positive affirmative messages are given by well-known people who have lost weight, given up smoking, alcohol or street drugs, or who have suffered poor mental health and shared their experiences.

Nursing associates are encouraged to use short health-promoting messages at every possible interaction with patients. 'making every contact count' (MECC) offers short suggestions to make small health improvements. Encourage your patients to walk, run or jog and remind them that it is difficult to smoke, drink and eat while exercising. You should direct your patients to the NHS website 'Change4Life', which offers a huge suite of advice on diet, exercise, mental health and other health promoting activities.

Chapter summary

This chapter has introduced you to the anatomy and physiology of communication, the nuts and bolts of how physiology supports verbal communication and the cognitive effort of interpreting sounds. We discussed how disorders can interfere with communication and examined strategies

(Continued)

that could be used to overcome barriers. We examined theoretical models of information exchange between the sender and receiver and how communication takes place, and discussed factors that influence the message. We then looked at interpersonal skills such as body language, and pitch and tone in speech, and how this influences communication. We also considered effective communication between healthcare professionals and used a case study to underpin the effects of poor communication. Lastly, we looked at communication in health promotion and examined the means of message used in the Covid-19 pandemic.

Activities: brief outline answers

Table 2.1 Physiological disorders that can act as barriers to communication

Cognitive disorders	Apraxia, Traumatic brain damage, dementia, learning disability, amnesia, delirium, Huntington's disease, aphasia, Parkinson's disease
Hearing and listening disorders	Perforated eardrum, Ménière's disease, glue ear, Otosclerosis, Cholesteatoma, Tinnitus, age related hearing loss, ADHD
Speech disorders	Lisp, Stammer, Stutter, Dysarthria, mutism, cleft palate, autism, nonverbal learning disorder, autism
Reading body language difficulty	Social-emotional agnosia, social anxiety disorder, autism, learning disability
Blindness	Also deaf-blind

Activity 2.2 Critical thinking (page 37)

James would adopt a transactional model of communication, where he receives the sender's message and the angry relative's statement and then processes the information. He then becomes the sender as he tries to deescalate the situation using cues, both verbal and nonverbal. His nonverbal body language would be open and relaxed to encourage the relative to calm herself. James can then address her issues. This is using a combination of communication and interpersonal skills to address the relative's concerns.

Activity 2.4 Communication (page 42)

Bethany asked Mrs Adebayo if she would give her permission to contact the care home where she lives to see if she can get her prosthetic leg brought into the hospital. Bethany called the home, who confirmed that Mrs Adebayo was correct and that a member of staff would bring the prosthetic in for her. They also apologised and said that when Mrs Adebayo was collected by ambulance staff she was very unwell and was not wearing her prosthetic. Bethany informed Mrs Adebayo and further informed the physiotherapy team about the missing information and the effect it had upon Mrs Adebayo.

Bethany stated 'As an advocate for my patients, it is important we truly listen to what they have to say, this could have had serious implications for Mrs Adebayo because the communication was so poor' (Nursing Associate Bethany Parker).

Activity 2.5 Work based learning (page 44)

Angie provided a reflective account of her experience:

The staff I worked with fed back to me about how I communicated during the procedure. Sometimes the words I used, or the way I inflected my voice, came across in a way that elicited a response from the patient and sometimes they would move/ nod their heads or try to talk back to me. Which in this circumstance could cause injury to patient if they were to move while the camera was down their oesophagus. I reflected on this, and decided I needed a more effective way to communicate to patients to preserve their safety, and I needed to be more self-aware of my word choices. In order to still reassure them, while maintaining their safety. I also needed to ensure that patients had a safe way of communicating their wishes during the test (i.e., if they wanted to withdraw consent for the test). Therefore, prior to procedures starting, I decided I would discuss with patients the importance of not speaking or moving their head or neck during the procedure, and explained the safety reasons for this while identifying that patients could raise their hand in the air as a way of communicating if they wished to stop the test.

It is important to me that I ensure my patients are safe and that they have a positive experience while in my care, and I strive to have effective communication in my daily practice.

Effective communication is important, especially in this instance, because I used communication as a distraction technique and offered patients reassurance throughout their procedures, helping them to relax and have a more positive experience of what is normally an uncomfortable test. Patients are usually very anxious about the test and the results prior, so it is important that they feel safe and as comfortable as possible while knowing that an alternative way to communicate their needs had been identified. Open and honest communication between multi-disciplinary team members is also important because it helps to promote safety of patients and it helped me to improve my self-awareness and communication skills to become a better nursing associate.

Nursing Associate Angie Blakey

Further reading

Myles Harris has written a book for the Understanding Nursing Associate Practice series of which this book is a part, detailing person-centred care in which he examines interpersonal skills in detail.

Harris, M. (2021) *Understanding Person Centred Care for Nursing Associates.* London: Sage.

Filiz Akkiline considers that the same gesture in diverse cultures may have a completely different meaning, and developing cultural competence is a means to avoid misunderstanding in communication.

Akkilinc, F. (2019) The body language of culture. *International Journal for Innovation Education and Research*, 7: 32–9. Found at www.researchgate.net/publication/335689301_The_Body_Language_of_Culture

Haran Ratna has also written extensively on effective communication in healthcare. This is a really worthwhile read, as so many mishaps in healthcare occur purely because of poor interdisciplinary communication.

Ratna, H. (2019) The importance of effective communication in healthcare practice. *Harvard Public Health Review*.

Useful websites

NHS Change4Life www.nhs.uk/change4life

NICE have developed a suite of patient decision aids, which are evidence-based, so that you can support patients to make informed choices. They can be found at

www.evidence.nhs.uk/search?om=%5b%7b%22ety%22:%5b%22Patient%20Decision%20Aids%22%5d%7d,%7b%22srn%22:%5b%22National%20Institute%20for%20Health%20and%20Care%20Excellence%20-%20NICE%22%5d%7d%5d

RCN (2019) Health literacy and teach-back: www.rcn.org.uk/.../health-literacy-and-teach-back

RCN (2019) Communication: www.rcn.org.uk/clinical-topics/patient-safety-and-human-factors/professional-resources/communication

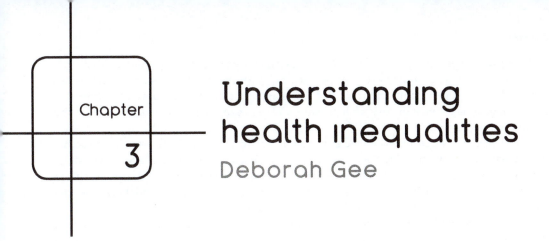

Chapter 3

Understanding health inequalities

Deborah Gee

Chapter aims

After reading this chapter you will be able to:

1.   understand the factors that lead to health inequalities;

2.   examine how inequalities are measured and reported within society;

3.   identify and discuss how unequal differences within society can influence the health and wellbeing of individuals;

4.   use the above knowledge to explain how inequality affects communities and populations.

Introduction

Why is there such a difference in life expectancy between people living just a few miles apart? For instance, people born in the London areas of Knightsbridge and Belgravia have a life expectancy of 93 years, but a few stops on the tube to Hammersmith and life expectancy drops to 79 years (life.mappinglondon.co.uk, 2021). In 2008, the London Health Observatory showed that if travelling east on the tube from Westminster, every two tube stops represented more than a year of life expectancy lost. These startling facts capture how health equalities can vary within small geographical areas. The differing dates of these studies also show that health inequalities persist in areas of deprivation. We will explore rural and urban deprivation further in the chapter.

Health inequalities are often defined as the unfair and avoidable differences in health across the population and between different groups in society. It is also suggested that health inequalities arise because of the conditions in which we are born, grow, live, work and age. These conditions influence our opportunities for good health, and how we think, feel and act and this shapes our mental health, physical health and wellbeing (NHS, 2020).

The broad social and economic circumstances which together influence the quality of the health of the population are known as the 'social determinants of health', which we were introduced to in Chapter 1. Work by Williams et al. (2020) highlights that the social determinants of health are often outside an individual's control. People living in the United Kingdom often experience systematic, unfair and avoidable differences in their health and the care they receive. All of which impacts upon their ability to live a healthy life across the lifespan. This chapter will discuss health inequalities, how health inequality is measured and the impact of inequality on marginalised groups. You are also asked to use your knowledge to undertake activities that reflect real life scenarios to check your understanding.

Understanding health inequalities

Within the context of healthcare, the term 'health inequalities' is often used to refer to differences that arise from socio-economic factors. These include income, work, housing and residence (other types of living accommodation, such as caravans and boats) with the inference that some people from a lower socio-economic group may deliberately choose more unhealthy ways of living (Naidoo and Wills, 2016). There are multiple interrelated causes of health inequalities, and, while the ability to access traditional health and care services play an important part in determining the health of a population, work by Marmot et al. (2010, 2020) and the WHO (2018a) suggests that access to traditional healthcare is not as important as the wider determinants. These would include the local environment, in addition to the conditions in which people are born, live and work.

Over the past few decades there have been a series of publications that have emphasised health inequalities and have made recommendations to support health and social care practitioners to manage the health of the population. These recommendations acknowledge the work of the NHS in the delivery of traditional healthcare services. In addition, the work emphasises that there should also be a co-ordinated delivery of a range of interventions, which are designed to tackle the underlying social, economic and environmental determinants across populations.

In 1977, the Labour government commissioned a report to investigate why there had been no reduction in the inequalities in health being experienced in society. In August 1980, the findings of the Inequalities in Health working group chaired by Sir Douglas Black, president of the Royal College of Physicians were published by the Department of Health and Social Security. This report provided detail to the extent of which ill health and death were unequally distributed among the population of the United Kingdom. The main findings made clear links between those living with unemployment, low income, poor education and substandard housing, and their health outcomes. Having concluded that these inequalities had been widening rather than diminishing since the establishment of the National Health Service in 1948, the report offered

37 recommendations which focused upon two main areas. The report recommended that the government should have policies aimed at reducing poverty and should increase spending on health education and prevention of illness.

By the time of its publication, the Labour government was no longer in power, having lost the general election to Margaret Thatcher's Conservative government in 1979. The Black Report was criticised and supressed (it was never printed) at the time. The Conservative government took no immediate actions to tackle the identified inequalities as suggested. This was due to a projected £2 billion cost of implementing the recommended health goals, tax changes and benefit increases.

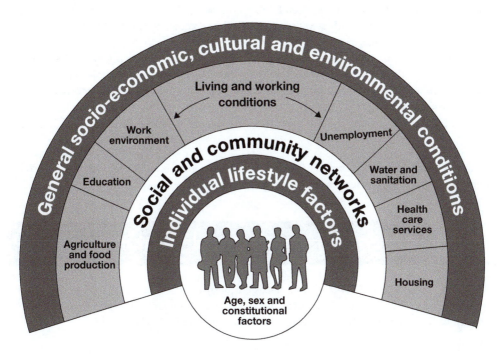

Figure 3.1　The determinants of health © WHO

The Health Divide Report (1987) was commissioned and produced by a group of professionals working independently to the government and led by Margaret Whitehead. The findings of the Health Divide Report concluded that the gap between health standards and social class had widened since the Black Report (1980). The Whitehead Report restated there was a direct link between health standards and social class. The Health Education Council campaigned on modifiable behaviours that are linked to health inequality such as alcohol, tobacco and food products. Unfortunately, the Conservative government dissolved the Health Education Council before it could formally publish its findings. The Acheson Enquiry (1988) also identified key areas of concern between social class and mortality rates. Margaret Whitehead and Göran Dahlgren produced the rainbow of inequalities in 1991 (see Figure 3.1), called the determinants of health, which maps the relationship between the individual, their environment and health. These reports collaboratively identified the causes of health inequalities as social, economic, cultural and political, thus actions to tackle these should also involve actions that take into account the social, economic, cultural and political factors.

Case study 3.1: George

George is aged 67 years old, and lives in Northeast England with his wife Sarah. George and Sarah have been married for 45 years and have two children. George worked in the shipbuilding industry for approximately 35 years until he was made redundant at the age of 52. George went on to have a series of temporary positions with other employers. Redundancy has had a huge impact upon his life and George has struggled for many years with his mental health.

In his early 60s, George developed Type 2 diabetes, this is currently managed with oral medications. Recently, George has been finding it increasingly difficult to manage his blood glucose levels. He walks with a walking stick and has known mobility issues due to his arthritic knees and spine.

George has been attending his GP surgery for his regular diabetes review and is noted to be significantly overweight. Blood tests have revealed he has raised cholesterol levels. George's GP has given him another medication to take, but it makes George feels nauseous and he does not take it.

Activity 3.1 now asks you to consider George's case study and some of the possible underlying medical and social reasons for his health problems.

Activity 3.1   Critical thinking

Using the case study, identify the health needs currently being experienced by George. Once you have identified these, can you make links to health determinants shown in Dahlgren and Whitehead's rainbow map that impact upon George's ability to live a healthy life.

An outline answer is given at the end of this chapter.

Thinking about George and his life over the last 40 years, there have been many significant changes in society. In the 1970s and 1980s, work was mainly heavy industry, mining, ship building, steelmaking, car manufacturing and factory production work. Although the hours were long, the work was secure and paid a reasonable wage. Usually, earnings were enough to buy a house, especially if someone was living in council accommodation and had the right to buy. House prices have risen exponentially, and home ownership is beyond the reach of many, leaving individuals and families at risk of high rent, poor-quality accommodation and the fear of eviction.

The report 'Tackling Health Inequalities' (2009) acknowledged that although the health of the worst off in England had improved since the 1988 Acheson Enquiry, the gap between the average and the worst off has not narrowed. The data presented showed persistent inequalities in income, educational achievement, literacy, child poverty, crime and unemployment. Even with some political commitment to improvement across these areas, it is clear that inequalities are deep-seated structures within society.

The Marmot Review (2010) went onto raise the profile of the wider determinants of health by emphasising the strong and persistent link between social inequalities and disparities in health outcomes. This review outlined a range of policy recommendations, some of which have been adapted and used as indicators of social determinants of health, health outcomes and social inequality.

These are the six priority objectives listed in the 2010 Marmot Review are:

1. *Give every child the best start in life.*
2. *Enable all children, young people and adults to maximise their capabilities and have control over their lives.*
3. *Create fair employment and good work for all.*
4. *Ensure a healthy standard of living for all.*
5. *Create and develop healthy and sustainable places and communities.*
6. *Strengthen the role and impact of ill health prevention.*

Many studies describe how it is not just access to healthcare provision that influences the health of individuals. They conclude that the social and economic factors often have a more significant impact on the health of the individuals, communities and populations. There have been repeated calls following the publication of the Marmot Review (2010) that government should tackle these issues as a matter of priority. To successfully address persistent health inequalities across society would require the political will to embark upon one of the most comprehensive and multifaceted programmes to tackle the underlying social determinants of health. In 2010, the Labour government did agree to make tackling health, social and educational inequalities a priority, and set a series of public health service agreement targets. However, with the change in government in May 2010 to the Conservative–Liberal Democrat coalition, this approach came to an end. The introduction of significant austerity measures, intended to reduce the national deficit, meant substantial cuts to funding for local authorities, reductions to the NHS budget (the Nicholson challenge) and the education sector, in addition to various restrictions being placed upon the welfare system.

Measuring inequalities

Although NHS England acknowledge the need for meaningful data as essential to providing the evidence base for effective healthcare delivery, there is also a need consider any implications of inequality.

Public Health inequalities are measured in different ways, however, the main broad measure of inequality is life expectancy. This is the difference in life expectancy between the most and least deprived areas of the UK. We looked at this at the beginning of the chapter using the London underground tube stations. Data findings published in 2020, show that the gap in life expectancy is widening, with average life expectancy for males and females living in the most deprived areas being 73.9 and 78.6 years, respectively. Whereas in the least deprived areas, the life expectancy for males is 83.4 years and for females it is 86.3 years. This most recent published data shows that the male life expectancy is less in more deprived areas, with males in the least deprived areas living on average 9.5 years longer (Gov.UK, 2020). According to the King's Fund, from 2011, increases in life expectancy slowed after decades of steady improvement, prompting much debate about the causes. The data published does not account for the mortality rates occurring due to the Covid-19 pandemic (Raleigh, 2021).

It has been noticeable that Covid-19 has affected lower socio-economic status people much more than white-collar workers. Many people employed in office-based jobs were furloughed and paid 80 per cent of their salary, or they could work from home. Service sector workers such as those working in social care, security, food production lines and retail were people who could not afford to self-isolate.

Despite the inequality in life expectancy being notably variable across the UK, the data still indicates that people living in more affluent areas are living longer than those in more deprived areas. Research work led by the King's Fund (2015) acknowledges that although the data is clear, we need to also consider the quality of life being experienced by those who may be living longer.

Williams et al. (2020) note that inequalities are ultimately about the differences in the care that people receive, and the opportunities they have had to live a healthy life across the life course. Between 2011 and 2019, those living in the most deprived areas are reported to spend nearly a third of their lives in poor health, compared to those living in least deprived who spend only a sixth, hence, not only do those living in deprived areas have the shortest lifespans, they also live more years in poor health (Raleigh, 2021).

Some populations have a shorter life expectancy than the general population. Research data shows that males with learning disabilities have shorter lives by 23 years (HQIP, 2019). Those in society affected by homelessness are also at significant risk with the average age of homeless males and females living 30 and 38 fewer years respectively than males and females in the general population (ONS, 2019b).

There are many deaths that are avoidable. These fall into two categories:

1. Preventable mortality: these deaths can be avoided through effective public health and **primary prevention** interventions.
2. Treatable mortality: these deaths would be avoidable through timely and effective healthcare interventions.

This is something that is also discussed in the work of the WHO (2013, 2018b), within their reports relating to the largely preventable non-communicable diseases, such as cancers, diabetes mellitus, chronic respiratory diseases and cardiovascular disease. All of these are causally linked to health inequalities. The Office for National Statistics (2020) report that in 2019, 80 per cent of all avoidable deaths fell into four main groups: cancers, respiratory diseases, circulatory diseases and substance misuse (drugs and alcohol). Cardiovascular, respiratory disease and lung cancer are reported as the main causes of death in those living in the most deprived areas of England (Gov.UK, 2020).

The Marmot Review update 'Health Equity in England: 10 Years On' (2020) found that improvements to life expectancy have stalled and have actually declined for the poorest 10 per cent of women. The review also found that there is a strong regional variation. The poorest in the northeast of England are worse off than the poorest in London. Marmot further states that 'Over the past decade there has been a significant shift in expenditure across government, moving from spending on the services and infrastructure that help people stay healthy, towards addressing problems that could be avoided in the first place' (healthfoundation.org, 2020).

Health literacy

Health literacy is defined by the World Health Organization as a 'The personal characteristics and social resources needed for individuals and communities to access, understand, appraise and use information and services to make decisions about health' (WHO, 2021c). Recent research by Public Health England tells us that between 43 per cent and 61 per cent of English working-age adults routinely do not understand health information. In the UK, 1.7 million adults read and write at or below the level of a nine-year-old and, critically, 43 per cent of adults do not understand written health information. Jonathan Berry (2016) gave examples that included a lady who thought her 'positive' cancer diagnosis was a good thing and couldn't understand why she wasn't getting better, and another lady who sprayed her inhaler on her neck because she had been told to 'spray it on her throat'. Nobody had checked whether she knew she had to open her mouth and inhale. He went on to say, 'Our system provides oral and written information to patients of such complexity that it far exceeds people's functional skills in language, literacy and numeracy, and therefore their ability to make sense of it and act on it'. Inadequate health literacy is associated with difficulties in understanding health information. Many people have limited knowledge of their own bodies and body functions, and the diseases that afflict it. This leads to lower medication adherence, which, in turn, contributes to poor health, risk of mortality, ineffective use of healthcare resources and increased health outcome disparities.

Nutbeam (2000) created three levels of health literacy:

1. *Functional: basic reading, writing and numerical skills used in a health context.*
2. *Interactive: advanced cognitive skills which allow the individual to conduct meaningful health conversations.*
3. *Critical: the individual can critically analyse information and use this to exert greater control over life events and situations.*

Providing information that is easily understood is a key health promotion activity. This allows the patient to give informed consent, participate in planning their own care and manage long term conditions. Also, communicating in a manner the patient feels comfortable with, and simple and clear language, gives patients the confidence to ask questions without feeling uncomfortable or stupid. Health Education England offer a toolkit to support you to support your patients and this can be found at: https://healtheducationengland.sharepoint.com/

Rural deprivation

Case study 3.2: Critical thinking

Tamsyn lives in the southwest of Cornwall, she and her two children are in rented accommodation and her children attend the local school. She and her children were born in the village and have strong local roots. The house she lives in needs remedial work as it is damp and does not have central heating. She has a coal fire in the lounge as a primary form of heating, with an expensive-to-run electric radiator in the children's bedroom. The village does not have a gas supply. Both children suffer from pulmonary ailments and have inhalers for asthma. They often take time away from school when they are unwell. The nearest hospital is 30 miles and three buses rides away. It takes 2 hours to reach the hospital by public transport and the cost is expensive. Tamsyn has a part-time job in the local shop and her wage is topped up with Universal Credit, which includes housing benefit. Tamsyn suffers from stress-related ailments and takes medication for anxiety and depression. She is frightened to complain to her landlord about the damp as she thinks her landlord will evict them and turn the house into a holiday home.

Activity 3.2 Reflection

Using knowledge you have gained so far, place Tamsyn's inequality characteristics into the following factors: health, social living, work and education.

Health	
Social living	
Working	
Educational	

Compare your answer with the one given at the end of the chapter.

The rural fringes of the UK are both attractive and deprived. Employment tends to be seasonal and based in the hospitality and agricultural sectors, both of which are poorly paid. Both sectors used to offer accommodation to offset the wage and to attract employees. Now, such accommodation is turned over to holiday makers. Rural deprivation is mainly hidden. May et al. (2020) noted that austerity compounds problems of rural poverty. Tamsyn's housing problem is exacerbated by rising house rental costs and the lack of either social housing or genuinely affordable housing. Eleven per cent of Cornwall's housing stock are second homes and average house prices have risen by 300 per cent in the last five years. May et al. also noted that urban dwellers live within 2.5 miles of a GP. Many rural households travel much further. The same applies to supermarkets and banks: 44 per cent of rural dwellers travel more than three miles to shop and access banking facilities. Small local shops tend to be 10–15 per cent more expensive and carry fewer goods. Tamsyn's village does not have a gas supply, so she suffers from fuel poverty. Fuel poverty considers households whose energy costs are higher than can be sustained by their income. She must buy smokeless fuel from the local shop and use an expensive method of heating the children's room to mitigate the damp.

The problem for calculating rural deprivation indices is that wealthy incomers skew the results. For example, six out of the top ten people on the *Sunday Times Rich List* live or have homes in Cornwall. Cornwall has a residential population of approximately 565,968 but this rises by an additional 850,000 in the summer months, and this places intense strain on the single Cornish hospital.

Urban deprivation

Urban deprivation is a standard of living that falls below that of the majority in a particular locale, area or society. Places suffering from urban deprivation have visible differences in housing, high unemployment, limited access to healthy food, few community resources and limited access to health facilities. Urban decay refers to run down, badly maintained houses, shuttered shops, empty factories, vandalised buildings and high levels of air and ground pollution.

Many of the factors in urban deprivation are historical, lack of town planning in the past led to narrow streets, which causes traffic congestion, which leads to poor air quality. Many post-war houses were of dubious build quality, especially council houses which were system-built, deck access houses, which are notorious for damp.

As traditional industries declined due to lack of government support, the export of manufacturing to low-cost Asian countries or changing market conditions, those who were able to migrated to where work was available. Leaving behind an area which became progressively poorer. High unemployment and higher crime rates ensure these areas remained deprived. Houses lose their value and eventually sell as 'buy to lets', which are poorly maintained. The concentration of low-income groups in deprived areas bring many social problems. Low property rental prices attract poorer immigrants, who are least likely to be offered loans and mortgages.

The net result of urban decay is that there is low investor interest to start up new industry in the area. People feel abandoned and become depressed. Children are less future orientated and have lower aspirations (with notable exceptions), lack of scholastic achievement means low-skilled, low-paid work. This is the engine that drives the cycle of deprivation or inherited poverty.

Health impacts of deprivation on individuals and families

The cycle of deprivation is what happens when people or areas suffer from a combination of linked problems such as unemployment, poor skills, low incomes, poor housing, crime, bad health and family breakdown. These problems are linked and mutually reinforcing, hence the cycle.

As we have discussed, poverty and ill health are closely inter-related. Poor people have little power to make changes and unequal power and opportunities play a pivotal role in creating an uneven distribution of social determinants of health. We know the causes of poverty are complex and entwined, and include unemployment, low-paid work, inadequate state benefits and lack of affordable housing. Here, they also intersect with disability, poor physical and mental health, lone parenting, being an unpaid carer, and being older and alone.

Within the cycle of deprivation is a health deprivation cycle. The significant association between poor physical and mental health and poverty is explained by the stresses associated with poverty. Having poor physical and mental health makes it difficult to find and keep work. Very few employers offer any degree of flexibility to accommodate periods of ill health.

A child born into poverty is likely to have a low birth weight which could impact on cognitive development. S/he is less likely to be breastfed and the mother is more likely to suffer from post-natal depression. As the child grows, s/he is more likely to suffer tooth decay, malnutrition, obesity and ultimately, diabetes and cardiovascular problems. Poor children also have a higher rate of accidents and accidental death. They also are 13 times more likely to die from unintentional injury (Watson and Lloyd, 2019). Gibson and Asthana (2000) make the correlation between low household income and poor educational performance. Child poverty can have a direct negative effect on children's social, emotional, developmental and cognitive outcomes. As the child grows into adulthood they are at risk of long-term and life-limiting illnesses. This accounts for poor life expectancy.

The effects of inequalities within marginalised groups

The research work undertaken by the King's Fund (2015) is a significant contribution to understanding social inequality. Researchers highlight evidence which shows that those from lower socio-economic groups and those with lower levels of educational attainment are not actively engaging with positive lifestyle choices. They note this as a public health concern given the variety of health education approaches and health campaigns active within the UK.

Activity 3.3   Critical thinking

Who do think falls into a marginalised group and what are the protected characteristics? And how do these groups of people have inequalities in accessing healthcare?

Jot down your thoughts and then compare them with Table 3.1.

There is also a lack of positive lifestyle choices across the lifespan, which indicates that the problems are persistent, complex and multifaceted. Therefore, there is a need to adopt a more holistic approach to addressing contemporary inequalities. It is quite demonstrable that people with lower socio-economic status engage in risk taking behaviours, such as tobacco use, alcohol misuse, poor diet, a lack of exercise and street drug use. These behaviours have persisted through generations (the cycle of deprivation), but it is not clear why. There are sociological and psychological explanations, but it seems a lack of future orientation also has a role. Low lifetime earnings give people less reason to plan for the future. Poor coping strategies for stress, such as comfort eating tend to be familial. Tobacco, street drugs and alcohol are used for relaxation when other means of escape are unaffordable.

The lower lifespan statistics include those with 'protected characteristics' from populations often defined as being part of 'health inclusion' groups. As explained earlier, they are at significantly higher risk of experiencing inequalities in accessing healthcare services (see Table 3.1). Their situation is summed up by Tudor's (1971) inverse care law: those most in need of attention by health services are often the least likely to receive that care.

Table 3.1 Inequalities in accessing health services experienced by people with protected characteristics and by health inclusion groups.

Protected characteristic	Inequality of access
Young people	There is evidence of service gaps for young people reaching adulthood particularly for those with complex needs. Young people with ADHD and autism can find it especially difficult to transition to adult mental health services that often do not offer specific services for their conditions.
Disabled people	Transport costs and long waiting lists can be barriers to equal access for disabled people. Breast screening, and contraceptive advice, smear tests are significantly lower for people with learning disabilities than in the general population.
Black and minority ethnic (BME) groups, including Gypsy, Roma, and Traveller (GRT) communities	Some Black and minority ethnic groups can have less access to healthcare services. Gypsy, Roma, and traveller communities face substantial barriers and have some of the lowest rates of healthcare access. Discrimination, lack of cultural awareness, literacy and language barriers can also create problems with access.
Religion and belief	Healthcare can be influenced by a person's religion and belief towards things such as abortion, contraception, and neonatal care. Specific views on dying, death and the afterlife are often influenced by religion. The religious beliefs of people are not always considered during care planning or when people attend healthcare settings. This can be considered a form of indirect discrimination and can have a negative impact on diagnosis and treatment, in addition to causing distress for patients and their families.
Lesbian, bisexual, gay and transgender (LBGTQ+) communities	Barriers to accessing services can be because of a lack of understanding of LGBTQ+ health concerns. Equality and diversity training for staff around the health needs of LGBTQ+ people can be lacking, often resulting in unsympathetic approaches to care.
People with alcohol and substance misuse needs	Stigmatisation and discrimination experienced by people who are dependent on alcohol or other substances have resulted in individuals not being accepted on to practice lists, and an inability to access medical care for conditions not related to their substance misuse.
Asylum seekers and refugees	Difficulty in accessing healthcare by these groups has been reported due to lack of awareness of entitlement, difficulties registering and accessing primary and community healthcare services, and language and literacy issues.
Carers	Evidence suggests that there is a lack of recognition of the caring role and the needs and issues related to caring within the health service. Failure to provide flexible appointment times, in addition to costs, waiting times, and transport and car parking difficulties, prevent carers from attending to their own health needs.

Information adapted from Institute of Health Equity (2018)

From examining this table and the activity you undertook (Activity 3.3) you will realise that stigma and discrimination pays a large role in barriers to access. As a nursing associate, you will understand how your non-judgemental attitude can have a positive influence in helping marginalised patients to feel accepted and respected. Supporting a marginalised individual will ripple through their community and encourage other to engage with health services.

New ways of working

In 2012, the Health and Social Care Act introduced the first legal duties for health bodies such as the Department of Health, Public Health England, Clinical Commissioning Groups and NHS England (the devolved nations of Scotland, Wales and Northern Ireland were required to introduce many of the provision of the act) which stated the need for such bodies to have due regard to reducing health inequalities between the various populations of England. The introduction of the Health and Social Care Act (2012) also brought about changes for the local authorities on Public Health Functions.

In response, Public Health England published 'Towards a Public Health Surveillance strategy for England' (2012). Public Health England suggested that effective **surveillance** and collection of data would be key in determining the needs of the population, stating that their vision was to offer world-leading surveillance services which provide a robust evidence base for decision making, and action-taking in respect of both acute and chronic diseases and health determinants. PHE stated that 'Surveillance will underpin the protection and improvement of health and service delivery, through outputs that are timely, accurate, accessible and meaningful to users of this information at the local, national and international level'. The systematic collection, analysis, interpretation and dissemination of data for a given population can help in ensuring that responses to specific identified areas of need are delivered at the right time, and in the most effective and equitable way. Essentially, if the various organisations that make up the NHS and individual staff members were to work effectively to reduce the health inequalities, this would ensure that everyone was given the same opportunities to lead a healthy life, no matter where they live or who they are.

NHS England acknowledges that there needs to be a significant improvement in the way healthcare professionals help people to live healthier lifestyles. A preventative approach was the starting point for the work that was carried out in the 'NHS Five Year Forward View' in 2014. That report addressed the need for a review of the structure primary and acute care services. It proposed an increased workforce with strong leaders to ensure that all NHS processes can meet the demand of the population with effective utilisation of the resources available.

This five-year forward view provided consensus relating to why change was required to make improvements and how to address the persistent inequalities within society. Acknowledgment of the need for change is echoed throughout and although there is a clear expression that it is within the power of the NHS to change, strong leadership is required to facilitate this change. It was noted that fragmented service provision could further disenfranchise the marginalised. There is also appreciation that success would be dependent upon a well-functioning social care system too. The current long-term plan (NHS, 2019a) builds on the need for integrated care, focusing on GP provision and strategies for mental health, maternity services and cancer care. The government have increased the NHS budget by three per cent for the next five years (approximately £20 billion). It should be noted that this plan is exclusively for the NHS. It does not include funding for social care.

The financial burden due to health inequalities in England also remain of concern. It is estimated that the increased use of NHS hospital and healthcare services from those in the most deprived areas is around an extra £4.8 billion each year. Health inequalities are also estimated to cost the UK between £31 billion and £33 billion a year in lost productivity and between £20 billion and £32 billion a year in lost tax revenue and higher benefit payments (PHE, 2021).

During the spring of 2021, the Conservative government published plans for the introduction of the Office for Health Promotion, which will be situated within the Department of Health and Social Care. The focus of the office is to lead work across government to promote good health and prevent illness, which impacts upon an individual's ability to live a healthy life across the lifespan. This will have the hopeful addition of reducing some of the financial burden placed upon the NHS.

Approximately 80 per cent of an individual's health outcomes are not connected to the healthcare they receive but are a direct consequence of the preventable risk factors such as diets, smoking and exercise. The Office for Health Promotion aims to build upon the work of Public Health England, leading on national efforts to improve the health of the nation by tackling public health issues, including obesity and nutrition, mental health across all ages, physical activity, sexual health, alcohol, and tobacco use (Gov.UK, 2021a).

The role of the nursing associate

Across the health and social care sector, there are staff shortages of approximately 220,000 workers and this is why the role of the registered nursing associate was created. You will become a trained and skilled healthcare professional with the opportunity to provide holistic care across all four fields of nursing: adult, child, mental health and learning disability. As a qualified nursing associate within health and social care, you will actively engage with public health issues and tackling some of the inequalities experienced by individuals, populations and communities. Your role will be supporting and empowering people and communities to exercise choice and take control of their own health decisions and behaviours by encouraging people to manage their own care where possible.

Promoting holistic health

Health promotion interventions are seen as a way of facilitating active engagement in order to safeguard the health and wellbeing of individuals in need. Historically, any interventions suggested by nurses or healthcare professionals were often undertaken without question. Patients would do as they were told and adopt what has been referred to as the 'sick role' (Parsons, 1951). More recently this relationship has become much more balanced with all nurses and healthcare professionals being required to work in partnership with individuals accessing healthcare. People are now more likely to want to be actively involved in all decisions about care.

Involving people in their care is complex, empowering them to take responsibility and manage their own health, and to encourage patients to making positive lifestyle choices can be challenging. As a qualified nursing associate, you should be able to effectively listen to and address the health concerns, and give informed advice to help patients make changes in their behaviours.

Health and healthcare practice is a holistic process. There is an expectation that all nursing associates working within healthcare practice will be able to address the healthcare needs of an individual using a biopsychosocial approach (Chapter 7). Holistic practice is the ability to consider the individual's needs in a variety of circumstances, and to include involvement of the person's family and wider social and community network.

Within healthcare practice, the essence of true holistic nursing is to tailor care to meet the needs of the patient. However, in order to meet the needs of others, there is an expectation that, as nursing associates, we are fully aware of ourselves. When addressing the issue of health inequalities, there is an expectation that we can distinguish between what is desirable and what is unacceptable practice.

Case Study 3.3 highlights the variations of opinion in why people from low-income families are more likely to have poor health and asks you to use your knowledge to decide which opinion you support.

Case study 3.3: Ruth

You are visiting a friend, Ruth. She is quite upset as she has had a disagreement with her mother. Ruth explains that she has been to visit her uncle George (Activity 3.1) and told her mother that George's diabetes was getting worse, but that George didn't like the new tablets he had to take. Ruth's mother said he was a silly old fool and only had himself to blame, if he ate better food, he wouldn't be so fat and he wouldn't have diabetes. Ruth told her mother that George couldn't afford better food.

Ruth knows you are a trainee nursing associate and asks you to tell her mother that people from low-income families struggle to adopt a healthy lifestyle.

Activity 3.4 now asks you to consider how you as a nursing associate would answer Ruth, who is right? Ruth or her mother?

Activity 3.4   Critical thinking

Give consideration to what you have learned so far about health inequalities, how would you advise both Ruth and her mother

An outline answer is given at the end of this chapter.

Activity 3.4 asks you to reflect upon Ruth and her mother's argument and to think about the knowledge you have gained by reading this chapter, the answer given at the end of the chapter highlights the complexity of social inequality and the varying perspectives that influence your work.

Chapter summary

This chapter has provided you with an overview of health inequalities. You have been introduced to some of the avoidable and unjust differences experienced by individuals, communities and populations when accessing healthcare. As far back as the publication of the Black Report in 1980, the unequal distribution of ill health, morbidity and mortality amongst society has been evident. The key links between those living with low income, limited education and poor housing and poor health outcomes is startling. Despite any number of commissioned reviews and reports, the persistent link remains. Marmot (2020) makes clear that there is still much work to be done. From the plethora of publications, the evidence is clear that potential solutions are available, however, there needs to a focused and sustained approach to implementing them.

Activities: brief outline answers

Activity 3.1 Critical thinking (page 52)

Reflecting upon the health inequalities George may have experienced across his life course, some of the issues you may have been able to identify could include the following:

- Exploration of data regarding mortality rates as a measure of the population health. You may have been able to identify that George has lived in northeast England which has a history of higher levels of deprivation. The links between those most deprived and health issues have specific links as made by Marmot et al. (2010, 2020).
- Links between George's educational attainment, employment and financial stability would also impact upon his ability to live a healthy life across the life course.
- The health issues noted include his mental health problems. It is reported that George has experienced poor mental health since his redundancy, which continued as he was unable to find secure work. The impact of mental health and the ability to live a healthy life across the life course for both George and his family are well documented.

- Obesity, raised cholesterol, mobility issues and Type 2 diabetes are all conditions that can have an impact upon a person's ability to live a healthy life. The detailed pathophysiology (see Chapter 6) of diabetes is well understood, with the evidence explaining that a large proportion of those experiencing Type 2 diabetes could reverse this with appropriate engagement with positive lifestyle choices, which includes diet and exercise.

Activity 3.2 Reflection (page 55)

Table 3.2

Health	Both children and Tamsyn have health related ailments predicated on their living conditions, but Tamsyn's fear of eviction prevents any improvements to the house and maintains her anxiety.
Social living	Tamsyn wants to stay in her home village and ensure the children have strong social roots in the community. The isolated rural community has barriers to access to healthcare due to distance to the local health facility and the cost of public transport.
Working	Tamsyn's access to employment is reduced with very little employment opportunities available without personal transport/childcare. Tamsyn could be no better off financially in low waged full-time employment if she had vehicle and child care costs, she would lose her benefits and still be trapped in poverty.
Educational	The children have reduced life chances due to poor health and frequent absences from education.

Activity 3.4 Critical thinking (page 61)

There is an ongoing academic discourse relating to this scenario and no simple either/or explanation. Explanations for health inequalities often focus upon the cultural/behavioural versus materialist/structural, and psychosocial explanations, which in turn suggests that the adverse environmental conditions across the life course can lead to ill health. As you have learned from reading this chapter, poverty and poor health education has a lifelong impact on people's abilities to make good choices. You might argue that people in lower socio-economic groups do not choose to be poor but they are poor as a result of structural barriers, or you might argue that poor people should take a more active approach to modifiable risks to health.

Further reading

To deepen your understanding of health inequality, read these reports:

1. Institute of Health Equity (2018) *Reducing Health Inequalities Through New Models of Care: A Resource for New Care Models*. London: University College London.

2. *Health Foundation/Marmot Review Ten Years On*, found at www.health.org.uk/publications/reports/the-marmot-review-10-years-on

3. Public Health England (2021b) *Inclusive and Sustainable Economies: Leaving No-one behind Supporting Place-based Action to Reduce Health Inequalities and Build Back Better*. London: PHE.

Useful websites

The following websites are useful to aid your research and understanding.

The King's Fund: www.kingsfund.org.uk

This is an independent organisation working to improve health and care in England, the website is rich in health information.

Public Health England: www.gov.uk/government/organisations/public-health-england

Currently provides information relating to the reduction in health inequalities and protection and improvement of the health and wellbeing of the nation. This function moves later in 2021 to the new Office for Health Promotion. The website is not currently functional, but you can read about it here: www.gov.uk/government/news/new-office-for-health-promotion-to-drive-improvement-of-nations-health

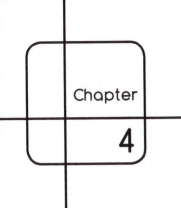

Chapter

4

Early years to adolescence and promoting good health outcomes

Deborah Gee

NMC STANDARDS OF PROFICIENCY FOR NURSING ASSOCIATES

This chapter will address the following platforms and proficiencies:

Platform 2 Promoting health and preventing ill health

2.5 Understand the importance of early years and childhood experiences and the possible impact on life choices, mental, physical, and behavioural health, and wellbeing.

Chapter aims

After reading this chapter you will be able to:

1. discuss the stages of brain development from birth to adolescence;
2. understand the importance of early childhood development and attachment;
3. identify the factors that can influence healthy childhood development;
4. critically examine the current key priorities in public health.

Case study 4.1: the Brown family

Carl and Hayley Brown have two children: Holly, age 15, and Emma, age 3.

Hayley found growing up extremely difficult, particularly throughout her pre-adolescent years, after witnessing years of excess alcohol consumption and domestic abuse between her parents.

(Continued)

Hayley married Carl when she was 18. When Hayley and Carl discovered they were expecting a child they were delighted. Holly was born, and they were settled as they only wanted one child. Hayley's second pregnancy with Emma was unplanned. When she discovered that she was pregnant with Emma, she found it extremely difficult to come to terms with expecting another child and began to drink alcohol secretly, which continued throughout the pregnancy. This led to rows when Carl found out, he felt increasingly angry and frustrated with her because he thought she was not accepting responsibility for her own actions.

Holly had experienced puberty when she was 13 years old and now wants to spend a lot of money on clothes, hair and makeup often saying that she feels that she is 'fat and ugly'.

Emma was born at 34 weeks gestation and struggled to feed. She was an unsettled and demanding baby and Hayley found this particularly challenging. In the first six months of Emma's life, Hayley would often rely upon her mother-in-law Sarah for help with Emma. This was not ideal as both Hayley and Sarah had opposing ideas on how to care for Emma, with Sarah often suggesting that Hayley should 'leave Emma to cry' when she was unsettled, telling Hayley that she 'must not spoil her'.

During Emma's 2½ year development check, the health visitor noted concerns regarding Emma's global development and referred her to the GP for further review. The GP referred Emma to the hospital consultant paediatrician for a specialist opinion. Hayley has found this difficult to accept, been reluctant to take Emma to the consultant paediatrician and missed two hospital appointments.

As we work through this chapter, we will revisit the family and discuss their problems in relation to childhood and adolescent development.

Introduction

This case study demonstrates the complex lives families have within society today. In practice we often work with people who have diverse personal, social and cultural backgrounds. There is an expectation as nursing associates that we have the ability to work with all persons across the life course addressing their physical and psychological needs, while adopting an appropriate evidence-based approach to practice.

Public health nursing is generally considered a specialist area of practice. The specialist community public health nurse (SCPHN) is a registered nurse who has undertaken an additional specialist qualification to work as either a health visitor, school nurse or occupational health nurse (NMC, 2018).

Other professionals may undertake periods of advanced training to support their practice when working in specialist areas of public health. However, as nursing associates we are also working within the NMC Code and there is a requirement to 'pay special attention to promoting wellbeing, preventing ill health, and meeting the changing health and care needs of people during all life stages' (NMC, 2018, p. 7).

This chapter will discuss the stages of childhood development from birth through to adolescence and beyond. We will begin by considering historical health improvements to child mortality and then discuss how a child brain develops. We shall consider the contributing factors that can impact upon a child's ability to experience a supportive and nurturing start to life. We will look at the work of critical theorists in childhood development. We will then go on to evaluate the impact of adverse events and targeted interventions to promote good health outcomes. We will then consider sexual identity, sexual health and emotional resilience. Throughout the chapter, there are activities for you to engage with and deepen your learning.

> *Children whose caregivers respond sensitively to the child's needs at times of distress and fear in infancy and early childhood develop secure attachments to their primary caregivers. These children can also use their caregivers as a secure base from which to explore their environment. They have better outcomes than non-securely attached children in social and emotional development, educational achievement and mental health. Early attachment relations are thought to be crucial for later social relationships and for the development of capacities for emotional and stress regulation, self-control and mentalisation. Children and young people who have experienced insecure attachments are more likely to struggle in these areas and to experience emotional and behavioural difficulties.*

(NICE, 2015)

A brief exploration of child mortality

Across the world there is clear evidence that a child being born today has a greater chance of survival than they would have done four decades ago. In 2019, the global under-5 mortality rates were around 59 per cent lower than they were in 1990. Data shows that on average 14,000 children under the age of 5 years died compared to the 34,000 who died in 1990 (IGME, 2020).

Data provided by ONS states that 2019 saw the lowest recorded number of infant and child deaths since records began (in 1980) with 3,297 deaths being recorded across England and Wales.

The report *The Best Start for Life* (Gov.UK, 2021b) highlights that babies are disproportionately in danger of abuse and neglect. In England, they are seven times more likely to be killed than older children. Around 26 per cent of babies (198,000) in the UK are estimated to be living within complex family situations, of heightened risk where there are problems such as substance misuse, mental illness or domestic violence.

During the period from 2014 to 2017, data also shows that there was a total of 368 Serious Case Reviews (SCR) involving the abuse or neglect of a child that has resulted in either the child being harmed or dying. Forty-two per cent of these cases were related to children aged under one year (Brandon et al., 2020).

Public health and local government departments have for many years provided a continuous stream of published research data. This has highlighted that the health inequalities that exist across the United Kingdom are a contributing factor to the mortality rates. These are unfair and preventable, given that they are often identifiable early in a child's life. This is concerning as children have no control over the inequality they are born into (Pearce et al., 2019). Poor childhood experiences are known to have a significant impact upon a child's attachment, resilience, readiness to learn and social behaviours, in addition to both physical and mental health.

Healthy child development

The healthy development of a child is dependent upon nurturing care. This would include the need for the child to experience a supportive environment where they feel safe and secure, have access to food and nutrition and receive responsive caregiving, with opportunities to learn. All of which are usually provided by parents, family members and positive social networks.

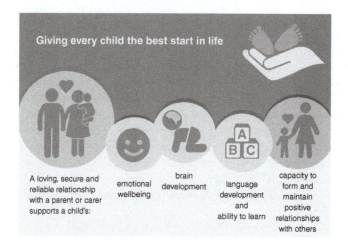

Figure 4.1 Giving every child the best start in life

(Public Health England, 2016, open source copyright)

A child's brain development

The development of a child through to adulthood involves a series of events. These span four different domains:

1. Biological: which incorporates physical growth and development of motor skills.
2. Cognitive: which refers to the processes leading to changes in memory, reasoning and problem solving.
3. Emotional: this aspect considers how a child experiences, manages and expresses emotions.
4. Social: which incorporates how a person understands themselves and how they relate to others.

Although the domains can appear to be individual, the process is holistic and therefore may involve the individual using developing skills that span across several of the domains at the same time.

Brain development

The brain can be divided into three regions (Chapter 4):

1. The brain stem which controls physiological processes such as respiration and digestion.
2. The cerebrum which consists of a left and a right hemisphere.

    (a) The left hemisphere controls movement and sensation on the right side in addition to processing language.
    (b) The right hemisphere controls movement on the left side and is connected to the capacity to identify visual and spatial relationships amongst objects.

3. The limbic system controls memory and emotional responses. There are three main parts to the limbic system to include the amygdala, the hippocampus and the cingulate gyrus.

Amygdala, hippocampus and cingulate gyrus

The amygdala is often referred to as the epicentre of the brain, the role of the amygdala is to control emotional reactions when responding to pain, fear or joy. When a baby is exposed to emotions, memories are formed. Memories are controlled by the hippocampus. Therefore, if the baby's memories are negative because of exposure to pain or fear, it will make it more difficult for anxious and stressed children to regulate their emotions (Menon et al., 2020). The cingulate gyrus is also involved in the processing of emotions and behaviour regulation.

Prefrontal and orbitofrontal cortex

The orbitofrontal cortex is the control centre, and it connects with social interactions. Through visual communication the baby decides on how to respond, for example, babies will seek out the attention of others, turn away when overwhelmed or freeze when they feel at risk. Up until the age of around three years, if social relationships are denied, the orbitofrontal cortex will not develop and will not recover.

The prefrontal cortex is the decision-making part of the brain helping younger children and adolescents to problem solve, and think about the consequences of their actions. It is one of the last regions of the brain to mature. The early years are critical to the foundations of brain development, however, the brain will still go through a period of remodelling before functioning as an adult brain. This process of remodelling takes place during adolescence and can continue until the child is in their mid-20s.

This process of remodelling involves the pruning away of unused connections while at the same time strengthening the developing connections. This process starts at the back of the brain, meaning that the prefrontal cortex is remodelled last. While the prefrontal cortex is still developing, teenagers may rely upon the amygdala to help them control their emotions, such as aggressive and instinctive behaviours.

Challenges between conception and two years of age

If a woman is suffering from excessive stress prior to conceiving and into the antenatal period, this can result in the baby's brain being flooded with cortisol for prolonged periods, which can be toxic to the developing brain. The foundations of the baby's mind are being put in place, optimum brain development is reliant upon positive experiences, even the most primitive experiences can influence and shape a baby's brain and can have a lifelong impact on the baby's mental and emotional health.

There is established evidence that a baby's social and emotional development is affected by their attachment to their parents. Hogg (2013) found that women experiencing perinatal mental illness can often fail to bond with their baby or be responsive to their baby's needs. International studies show that when a baby's development falls behind the norm during the first years of life, they are more likely to fall even further behind in subsequent years than to catch up with those who have had a better start (Gov.UK, 2021b).

Early relationships set the sensor for later control of a stress response. Research has shown that antenatal maternal stress is associated with a range of mental health problems in children such as attention deficit hyperactivity disorder (ADHD), anxiety and conduct disorders (Tuovinen et al., 2021).

Activity 4.1   Research and communication

Research the main factors relating to successful brain development.

If you had been working with Hayley and Carl's family when Emma was a baby, what would you have advised Hayley regarding her mother-in-law's advice?

What does the current evidence-based research say regarding the point of 'leaving Emma to cry' and that Hayley 'must not spoil her baby'?

How might this approach impact the holistic development of Emma?

Read these two pieces and compare your thoughts with the answer at the end of the chapter:

1. Ayten Bilgin and Dieter Wolke (2020). Parental use of 'cry it out' in infants: no adverse effects on attachment and behavioural development at 18 months. *Journal of Child Psychology and Psychiatry*; doi: 10.1111/jcpp.13223
2. www.nhs.uk/conditions/baby/caring-for-a-newborn/soothing-a-crying-baby/

An outline answer is given at the end of this chapter.

Attachment theory is now considered the 'gold standard' for assessing children's relationships with their caregiver. So, let us now turn to the theories and theorists.

Theorists

John Bowlby – Developing attachment

Psychologist and psychoanalyst John Bowlby was born in 1907. Throughout his career the focus for his work was around early childhood attachment, and how this would influence both the physical and psychological development of an individual. Throughout his work, Bowlby proposed that attachment bonds were formed using the five innate behaviours of sucking, looking, cuddling, smiling and crying.

Bowlby believed that attachment developed through four distinct stages. The first stage is pre-attachment, taking place between birth and two months, where he highlighted that babies show marked preferences for a human stimulus. His research demonstrated that babies wanted to see faces not objects.

The next stage is where the attachments are made. The baby interacts and wants to engage in taking turns. At times throughout this stage, infants may show a distinct preference for their main caregivers.

The period between seven months and two years is suggested to be a critical period where babies show they have formed strong attachments. These attachments are usually made with one person who is their primary caregiver. Following this, the infant will often display signs of having formed a relationship which leads to the final stage; a goal-corrected partnership where from around the age of two years a baby will cry to summon their primary care provider, showing the development of a basic relationship.

The hypothesis of John Bowlby's work was based upon the belief that an infant's attachment was an 'all' or 'nothing' type of situation. The conclusions Bowlby made as a result of his attachment theory work were that all children require a stable relationship with their mother or primary care giver.

Mary Ainsworth - Measuring attachment

In 1969, Mary Ainsworth and her assistant Barbara Wittig acknowledged the work of Bowlby but identified that his work was based upon research undertaken retrospectively on the childhood experiences.

Developing the Strange Situation Procedure (SSP), Ainsworth produced a measured way of observing young children which allowed them to show exactly how they were feeling. Children were observed in a controlled environment through a one-way mirror during a series of circumstances that involved the parent, child and a stranger being visible and available to the child.

This approach allowed Ainsworth to investigate the security of attachment in the two-year-old across four different categories: separation anxiety, willingness to explore, stranger anxiety and reunion behaviours.

This work resulted in Ainsworth believing that there are three distinct attachment styles secure, ambivalent and avoidant (see Figure 4.2). In 1990, Main and Solomon added a fourth attachment style of disorganised.

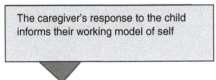

Positive and loved	Rejected	Angry and confused
Secure	Avoidant	Resistant

Figure 4.2   Styles of attachment

Bowlby and Ainsworth are just two researchers and theorists, Activity 4.2 now asks you to undertake some further reading to enhance your knowledge. We will return to Erikson further in the chapter.

Activity 4.2   Research

Earlier discussion relating to the work of John Bowlby and Mary Ainsworth have linked the theories of attachment to young children.

Undertake some additional research around the work of Erik Erikson (1902–1994) relating to psychosocial development, Jean Piaget (1902–1994) relating to cognitive development and moral psychology and David Elkind (1931–) relating to adolescent egocentrism. Jot some notes down and compare your writing with the statements at the end of the chapter.

An outline answer is given at the end of this chapter.

Developing a good understanding of child development theory will support your practice, the biopsychological development of children can give an indication of how well (or otherwise) a child will react to life's challenges. Poor coping strategies developed during childhood and adolescence can influence how that child will react to challenge as an adult.

Factors that can influence healthy childhood development

Adverse Childhood Experiences (ACEs)

There are three direct and six indirect experiences that have an impact on childhood development. The more adversity a child experiences, the more likely this will impact upon their developing brains.

Evidence suggests that children who are exposed to four or more ACEs are more likely to engage in risk taking behaviours and find it difficult to make positive changes.

Table 4.1 Adverse events

Domestic Violence	Verbal Abuse	Physical Abuse
Sexual Abuse	Parental Separation	Mental Illness
Alcohol Abuse	Drug Use	Incarceration

Information taken from the Centre for Public Health (2016)

The prevalence of Adverse Childhood Experiences

The initial concerns for a child with exposure to four or more ACEs are clearly linked to the developing brain. The impact of non-genetic influences can trigger an allostatic state which interrupts a child's ability to maintain a stable stress response and therefore will have an impact upon the function of the hippocampus and the amygdala (Sun et al., 2017).

ACEs can also result in physical damage to the child, such as bone fractures. There is an increasing amount of research, however, that suggests that the child will also experience increased levels of gastrointestinal problems, asthma and other somatic complaints.

Lower levels of school attendance resulting in poorer levels of educational attainment and increased antisocial and violent behaviours are undoubtedly part of the life course that connects childhood adversity with long term adult ill health (Bellis et al., 2018).

Mothers who have experienced ACEs including maltreatment and exposure to household stressors are more at risk of maternal physical and mental health problems during their lifetime (Braungart-Rieker et al., 2016). Repercussions of this altered state can result in the person adopting antisocial and health-harming behaviours.

As adults, the consequences for those behaviours are that those who have experienced more than four ACEs in their life will be twice as likely to smoke, six times more likely to use alcohol to excess and twice as likely to develop conditions such as cancers and heart disease (Bellis et al., 2018).

Although research has demonstrated that adversity may transfer from one generation to the next in the form of abuse, neglect, or poor socioemotional health (Sun et al., 2017), it is important to note that not all children will be impacted by ACEs, even if their parent was exposed to ACEs themselves.

In professional practice evidence-based prevention and early intervention can make a difference to the child's lifelong health and wellbeing (PHE, 2015). These will also help break the cycle of disadvantage experienced and improve the long-term outcomes for future generations.

Table 4.2   Estimated changes with effective prevention

Reduces underage sex	Reduces unintended pregnancy in teens	Reduces tobacco use	Reduces use of street drugs and cannabis	Reduces binge drinking
Reduces use of Class A drugs	Reduces victim of violence	Reduces violence perpetration	Reduces likelihood of incarceration	Reduced likelihood of diet related ailments

Information taken from the Centre for Public Health (2016)

Activity 4.3   Critical thinking

Using Case Study 4.1: the Brown family

Within the case study Hayley has experienced difficulties throughout her life in particularly throughout infancy and her adolescent years. Hayley witnessed years of excess alcohol consumption, substance misuse and domestic abuse between her parents.

Consider the detail within the case study, in particular, the life course events that have been experienced by Hayley. What specific links can you note to Adverse Childhood Experiences?

What are the potential consequences of Hayley's exposure to ACEs and for her own children?

An outline answer is given at the end of this chapter.

Hayley's older daughter Holly is now transitioning through adolescence, now let us look at how her experience of family discord (ACEs) can impact her successful transition.

Childhood to adolescence and beyond

As young people transition between childhood and on into adulthood, they experience a range of physical, behavioural, social and emotional changes. The onset of adolescence is the time a young person experiences the hormonal changes linked to puberty. It has been described as a predictable period where there are significant changes in the biological, cognitive, social and emotional systems. How a young person responds to these changes can be influenced by their previous life events (Ogden and Hagen, 2019). Adolescents come under the influence of their peers, social media and broadcast media. Media portrayals can influence behaviours (both socially acceptable and unacceptable). Activity 4.4 asks you to explore this further.

Hopkins (2010) suggests that young people are always under scrutiny within the population and can often be stereotyped or find themselves marginalised within society. All of which will have an impact upon their ability to experience positive healthy stages of development.

Activity 4.4   Research

Choose a selection of newspapers, magazines and digital publications from over the past month where the focus is on young people. What sort of things are being portrayed around the young person? How much of the information is known to be factual? What stereotypes of young people are being reinforced?

As your answers will be based around your personal research no outline answers are offered.

A young person's lifestyle choices and health behaviours are greatly influenced from around the age of 10 years. From the research you undertook for Activity 4.4, did you note media promoting physical activity to reduce obesity? It is well documented that physical activity declines during this period with one in four children aged between 11 and 15 years now being classified as obese (Hagell and Shar, 2019).

Public Health England (2021c) reports that nearly one third of children between 2 and 15 years are overweight. There is a notable increase in children becoming obese at a younger age and remaining obese for longer. Children living with obesity are more at risk of having lifelong health issues into adulthood such as Type 2 diabetes, musculoskeletal conditions or mental health conditions, such as depression.

The economic cost of obesity is a significant concern to the National Health Service with the reported costs being in excess of the national spending on the police, fire service and the judicial system combined. During the period from 2014 to 2015, this was estimated at around £5.1 billion.

The UK government have acknowledged that the challenges around obesity are a public health concern. In 2016, the *Childhood Obesity: A Plan for Action* was launched. This plan was focussed upon a multi professional approach to making food and drink healthier in addition to supporting healthier choices for children and young people (Gov.UK, 2016).

This work was followed two years later with the intent of ensuring reductions in the amounts of sugar contained within the common food's children eat (Gov.UK, 2018). Activity 4.5 asks you to consider different attitudes to food between older people that you may care for and younger people. Before answering this question, you could read Chapter 6 to inform your thinking.

Activity 4.5   Critical thinking

Within the UK it is evident that there are significant concerns relating to the issues of obesity and despite a continuous drive to tackle the issues and reduce the obesity crisis, the problem continues to worsen.

Consider the food lifestyle behaviours within the population that you nurse. Ask your patients about differences in attitudes towards food during the 1970s and today, how would older people reply?

How have we reached the point of concern we have in society?

An outline answer is given at the end of this chapter.

Twitter recently ran a survey asking the over 60s if they had access to snacks when they were children. Almost all replied that they did not. Activity 4.5 asked you to engage in your own investigations. What did you find?

In the past, people died from the diseases of poverty. Now, we die from the diseases of affluence. However, there are arguments that healthy food is more expensive than 'junk' food. It takes time and education to plan and cook cheap nutritious meals. People live busy lives, and either are too tired to cook from scratch or do not have the knowledge or facilities to do so. Most older people will tell you that snacks (fizzy pop, crisps, sweets) were an occasional treat, not daily occurrences.

Approaches to promote good health

In 2016, Public Health England set out their strategic four-year plan. This built upon the past successes from the NHS Five Year Forward View (NHS, 2014) and 'From Evidence into Action' (PHE, 2014). This work outlined the specific detail of the work that was necessary to improve population health and reduce inequalities.

The plans were bold, and the suggestion was that a targeted multi-agency approach would allow England to become the first country in the world to significantly reduce childhood obesity (PHE, 2016).

In 2019, the strategic plan was superseded and replaced by Public Health England Strategy 2020 to 2025. This more recent publication provides detail of the top ten priorities and the proposed plans for moving forward.

The earlier strategic plan was about targeted interventions linking specifically to the incidence and **prevalence** of health issues within populations across England. The new strategy adopts a different approach, where the focus of priorities is linked to the need to protect people, and to ensure that they are able to live longer in good health.

With a notable 19-year difference between the number of years spent in good health between the poorest and most affluent areas of society, it is important to recognise that the need for change starts with children and young persons. Poor health choices lead to long term health conditions, which in turn contribute up to 40 per cent of those experiencing poor health leading to early death. One of the biggest risks are what and how much we choose to eat (PHE, 2019). The following lists the ten target areas identified by PHE for action in the years 2020 to 2025.

1. *Smoke-free society*
2. *Healthier diets, healthier weight*
3. *Cleaner air*
4. *Better mental health*
5. *Best start in life*
6. *Effective responses to major incidents*
7. *Reduced risk from antimicrobial resistance*
8. *Predictive prevention*
9. *Enhanced data and surveillance capabilities*
10. *New national science campus.*

(PHE, 2019)

Activity 4.6. asks you to use this information and identify in what way these targets relate to your area of practice.

Activity 4.6   Evidence-based practice and research

Access the *PHE Strategy 2020–25* (PHE 2019) and consider how the ten target areas may link with your current area of practice as a nursing associate.

Read the report here: https://assets.publishing.service.gov.uk/government/uploads/system/uploads/attachment_data/file/830105/PHE_Strategy__2020-25__Executive_Summary.pdf

Examine the examples given and consider what approaches you can adopt within your practice linking directly to the targeted priorities listed?

As your answers will be based around your personal experiences in practice no outline answers are offered.

How many of the targets were you able to say linked to your area practice, and from the examples given, is there anything you can adapt in your practice?

Resilience: a way to help?

There are many things that can influence the child during adolescence, Holly wants to buy clothes and make up as she considers herself 'fat and ugly'. Young people's self-concept develops and differentiates, as does their does self-esteem. Their self-esteem varies under challenge, so when Carl and Hayley argue in front of her, she becomes distressed and introverted. Remember the research you did in Activity 4.2 and Erikson's fifth psychosocial task of identity versus role confusion. Holly feels that make-up and clothes will help her present a more acceptable identity to her friends, and to help her form romantic relationships. However, there is ample research which shows that low self-esteem increases the risk of developing depressive symptoms during adolescence. Sadly, there are significant variations of the support available across the United Kingdom, and this can potentially influence the whole of life outcomes. Activity 4.7 asks you what other social and cultural behaviours can impact on an adolescent's developing identity.

Activity 4.7   Critical thinking

As a nursing associate working with families across the life span, what social and cultural behaviours do you think may have an impact upon a child going through adolescence.

A model answer is given at the end of this chapter.

How many from the list given in the model answer did you think about? Researchers have found that children and adolescents with learning disabilities have higher rates of poor mental health and behavioural problems. Learning disabilities, such as dyslexia, dyspraxia, hyperactivity disorder, attention deficit disorder (ADD), autism and Asperger's syndrome often result in low self-esteem, which can cause depression and other poor mental health issues, which, in turn, can lead to poor coping mechanisms such as substance misuse.

Marmot (2020) continues to reinforce the links between inequalities within society and the poor health outcomes for the population. One of the suggested areas of focus to tackle some of these ongoing issues is the inclusion of work to build resilience.

Resilience is described as the ability to 'bounce back', this is not an innate feature of some peoples' personalities and those who experience inequalities within society are thought to be least likely to have the resources to build resilience.

Those who are resilient often see more positive outcomes, although it would be wrong to assume that those who are resilient will remain unharmed. People with high-risk backgrounds often see poorer outcomes than those who come from more low-risk backgrounds even if they have less resilience.

Four actions to increase resilience are to:

- increase the achievements of students;
- support children and young people through life transitions;
- encourage healthy lifestyle behaviours;
- promote improved interpersonal relationships.

Those who are resilient do well despite adversity, although it does not imply that those who are resilient are unharmed – they often have poorer outcomes than those who have a low-risk background but less resilience. By diversifying achievement criteria, non-academic students can feel a sense of self pride, helping children through transition such as from one school to another. Children entering senior school often suffer declines in self-esteem and have unaddressed worries about bullying and coping academically. Some senior schools have developed a buddy system, where an older school child supports a new entrant with such things as school geography and signposting to staff help when the 'newbie' is feeling overwhelmed. Evidence shows that by supporting children to develop resilience could contribute to healthy behaviours, higher qualifications and skills, better employment, better mental wellbeing and a quicker or more successful recovery from illness (Allen, 2014).

Disease screening: children with disabilities

In England, there are approximately 21 million screening tests carried out each year. This includes more than 600,000 newborn babies who are screened for 15 congenital disorders (PHE, 2019).

Disabled children and those who have long term conditions are more likely to experience disadvantage and harm. Ninety per cent of parents with a disabled child report that they felt their child did not have the same opportunities as a child who was non-disabled (Sense, 2016).

Parents of disabled children often report being physically and emotionally exhausted. They often feel isolated and lonely. The lack of understanding and negative attitudes often noted from friends and family, and from members of the public, can often feel like they are in a constant battle (Action for Children, 2017).

Research over the past decade has concluded that those children with disabilities and long-term conditions are often overlooked (DH, 2012). In 2019, the NHS stated that the aim was to ensure that, by 2028, all children and young people would have better physical and mental health. They suggest that this would be accomplished with the provision of a seamless and more integrated service between health and social care sectors. Achievement of this would require an appropriately trained and skilled workforce that would be able to listen, respond and meet the needs of those living with disability and long-term conditions (NHS, 2019a). As part of your nursing associate career, you may be supporting parents when they are given the news that their child has a disability or long-term condition. You can explore this further in Activity 4.8. Make a note of your thoughts.

Activity 4.8   Evidence-based practice and research

Hayley is clearly struggling with a possible diagnosis of disability or long-term condition for Emma and is hoping she will just grow out of her developmental delays. Parents often experience shock and denial, and feelings of anger and guilt.

As a nursing associate working with the families who receive this type of news, what would be the knowledge that you need to underpin your professional practice?

What skills do you feel you would need to use to support families in this situation?

An outline answer is given at the end of this chapter.

It is possible that Hayley feels guilty that her drinking while pregnant has had an impact on Emma. She could be frightened that she will be blamed by Carl, and this could have a devastating impact on their marriage. She may also be right that Emma's delays are maturation issues rather than evidence of an ailment.

Sexual health and sexual orientation

Throughout the transition to adulthood, the child will develop a sense of sexual identity. The process is often complex and greatly influences the behaviours of young people.

In 2021, the ONS reported that 2.7 per cent of the population had identified themselves as lesbian, gay or bisexual the largest rate in any age group was that of the 16–24-year-olds.

Although 1.4 million people aged over 16 years in the UK identified as lesbian, gay or bisexual, this figure could be higher as many respondents reported 'other' or 'did not know' as their response (ONS, 2021).

Sexual orientation and gender identity are distinct, and within the UK the availability of data is limited. For example, there is no specific data relating to exactly how many young people would identify themselves as transgender. The Government Equalities Office (2018) have attempted to provide a tentative estimate and suggest this would be somewhere around 200,000–500,000 in total, at this point there has been no attempt to offer a breakdown by age.

Work published by the Association for Young People's Health reports that 16 years is the average age for sexual intercourse. The use of contraception is something that many young people consider, with estimates of around 85 per cent of those engaging in intercourse between the ages of 16 to 24 years reporting the use of contraception the last time they had sex.

The use of condoms was the most common method in the younger age group, used by 61 per cent of the boys and 57 per cent of the girls. The contraceptive pill was the second most common method, followed by the morning after pill (emergency contraception) or another method (AYPH, 2019).

Emotional wellbeing

Public Health England's strategic plan (2016) reports that 50 per cent of mental illness experienced by adults began before they reached the age of 15 years. At that time, it was estimated that 695,000 children aged between 5 and 15 years had been diagnosed with a clinical mental health problem. The 2019 data suggested that at least one in six adults would have experienced a common mental health disorder such as depression or anxiety in the previous seven days.

The negative impact on a person's quality of life is estimated to cost society around £105 billion each year to manage. The life expectancy of a person with serious mental health problems is thought to be approximately 20 years less than someone without mental health issues within the general population.

Suicide is recorded as the leading cause of death for people between the ages of 10 and 34 years.

Public Health England (2019) have noted that there needs to be parity between the approaches to addressing mental health and physical health, with a greater emphasis on those who are most disadvantaged and living with long-term mental health problems.

Included within the identified ten priorities throughout 2020–2025, Public Health England have outlined a series of approaches to include providing advice on evidence-based preventative interventions to national and local government, academic institutions and voluntary community partners.

Chapter summary

This chapter has focused upon the different stages of childhood brain development from birth to adolescence. The individual factors that can have either a positive or negative impact upon healthy childhood development have been explored in addition to identifying some of the key public health priorities and targeted interventions.

Working within the NMC Code (NMC, 2018) you are required to promote wellbeing and meet the challenging care needs of all people throughout the life course and therefore all nursing associates need to ensure that they have the underpinning knowledge and skills to meet the needs of those who are most at risk and vulnerable within society.

Activities: brief outline answers

Activity 4.1 Research and communication (page 70)

Emma is a child. She cannot survive without help. She has basic needs, food, warmth, love and stimulation, and is dependent upon Hayley for everything. If Emma receives the care she needs from Hayley, she will develop a sense of trust using her positive cognitive, emotional and social skills. Professor Dieter Wolke said that his research shows there is no impact of 'leave to cry' on a newborn's development and attachment. However, differential responding means that babies were only left to cry for short periods initially, and longer cry duration periods as the infant got older. Unlike the NHS webpage, the researchers do not give the reasons for baby crying (hunger, pain, discomfort, need for reassurance). Trust in the caregiver to meet the babies need is established early after birth. Wolke's research conflicts with previous research undertaken by psychologist Dr Penelope Leach on infant neuroscience. Leach (2011) stated that denying a response can have long-term emotional consequences.

The issue of trust will have a significant impact upon the ability for her to develop relationships with others particularly in the young adult stage. The development of an intimate and loving relationship is reliant upon trust. If one of the people in that relationship has difficulties in placing trust in others this will impact upon the ability to share and develop loving relationships.

Activity 4.2 Research (page 71)

Psychosocial theory - Erik Erikson (1902-1994)

Erikson suggests that there is plenty of time across the lifespan for personal development, with his work placing an even greater emphasis on the impact an individual's culture and society will have on them. In the development of his eight stages model, Erikson believed that at each stage there is a psychosocial crisis with either a positive or negative outcome.

He suggested that those whose experiences that result in positive outcomes will be able to develop a positive healthy personality with a good sense of self, and those who fail to complete each of these stages effectively will result in a negative outcome and the individual may experience a sense of failure bringing an increased feeling of loss in the development of their identity and self-esteem. If this happens, Erikson highlights the increased risk of the individual not being able to contribute fully to society.

Jean Piaget (1902-1994)

Piaget had four stages of cognitive development. Piaget believed that intelligence was fixed at birth and that children would learn through experiences using a process of schemas they develop in order to shape their perceptions, cognitions and judgements of the world. Piaget believed that this approach provided the adolescent to have a reasoned scientific approach to complex situations.

David Elkind (1931-)

Elkind's work is based upon the work of Jean Piaget relating specifically to the formal operational stage. Elkind suggests that up until the age of around 15–16 years adolescents are preoccupied with themselves. This egocentrism leads them to also believe that others in society are equally as preoccupied with their self and their appearance as they are. Elkind also notes that the adolescent will perceive themselves to be in a position where they will not experience any misfortune themselves, for example, things like sex without contraception will never result in them becoming pregnant.

Activity 4.3 Critical thinking (page 73)

Adverse childhood experiences can include maltreatment in addition to exposure to household stressors. These traumatic events that occur in childhood can include the experiencing or witnessing of domestic violence, having a family member attempt or die by suicide, exposure to substance misuse from a parent or both parents, exposure to the parent experiencing significant mental health problems, parental divorce or separation.

Throughout Hayley's life she was exposed to several of these factors. Research indicates that exposure to these events could have had a detrimental impact upon Hayley's development and may have impacted upon her ability to build resilience.

A mother's experiences of childhood ACEs is significantly associated with substantial risks for their own children. This lack of a supportive secure attachment for Hayley throughout her formative years has resulted in the repeat of some of the behaviours learned from her formative years such as excessive alcohol consumption while pregnant, which was witnessed by Holly.

Activity 4.5 Critical thinking (page 74)

In the 1970s, there were far fewer children who were obese. Children rarely had snacks between meals. If they were offered anything it would most likely have been an apple, rather than crisps or chocolate.

Takeaways, such as chips and pizza, were a rare treat. Children received a nominal amount of pocket money and often only used this to buy their sweets once a week. Children's play was much more active: walking or cycling instead of being driven, playing football or long rope skipping in the street, etc.

Activity 4.7 Critical thinking (page 76)

Some of the elements you may have been able to identify may include:

Disability; learning difficulties; peer pressure; divorce and parental conflict; parents going to prison; chronic illness; cultural differences; social differences; sexuality; gang culture.

Activity 4.8 Evidence-based practice and research (page 78)

The way in which parents are given the diagnosis for their child can often have an impact upon their ability to adjust to the situation and make appropriate adjustments to ensure that they are able to address the ongoing health needs for their child.

There are barriers for both the family and the professional when in a breaking-bad-news situation. Families often report the use of poor communication skills by the professionals. They can feel like they have been given too little or to much information and it is often not offered in a language that they can use.

The professional can sometimes have little or no experience in these situations and can often feel unprepared for the event. Not feeling able to respond to the families' emotions or behaviours following a diagnosis can leave the professional feeling inadequate in supporting the family.

Depending upon the age and capacity to understand, the child has the right to be involved in decisions about their health, and parents should be asked if they wish the child to be present when the news is given.

It is important to remember that children will often provide a response based upon the response of their parent and sometimes and this can bring additional challenges. For example, if the parents do not want the child present for a reason, you would need to ensure that the child was not left alone when the news is being given to the parents.

It is important never to assume what the initial responses of parents or family members may be. These can be complex and can often be influenced by cultural or familial factors (Glasper et al., 2015).

Further reading

As a registered nursing associate, you need to have a good grasp of the legal framework in which you deliver care. You should read *The Children Act* 1989, 2004, the *UN Convention on the Rights of the Child* (1989, 1991), *Getting It Right for Children, Young People, and Families* (DH, 2012) and *The Children and Families Act* 2014.

You could do some background reading: Chapter 3: Legal and Professional Issues.

Benbow, W. Jorden, G. Knight, A and White, S. (2019) *A Handbook for Student Nurses*, 3rd edition: introducing key issues relevant for practice.

You can also read Chapter 3: Healthcare Ethics and the Law and Chapter 5 Inclusivity in Care in Harris, M. (2021) *Understanding Person Centreed Care*. London: Sage.

Further reading can be found in Chapter 13 which details protecting vulnerable children and Chapter 14 which covers additional needs and challenging behaviours.

Rowe, G., Ellis, S., Graham, K., Henderson, M., Barnes, J., Counihan, C. and Carter-Bennett, J. (2020) *A Handbook for Nursing Associates and Healthcare Practitioners*. London: Sage.

Useful websites

The following websites are useful to aid your understanding.

The King's Fund (www.kingsfund.org.uk)

This is an independent organisation working to improve health and care in England.

The Department of Health and Social Care: Department of Health and Social Care – GOV. UK (www.gov.uk)

Providing latest updates on health and social care issues to help people live more independent, healthier longer lives.

Public Health England: Public Health England – GOV.UK (www.gov.uk)

Provides information relating to the reduction in health inequalities and protection and improvement of the health and wellbeing of the nation.

The Office for National Statistics: Office for National Statistics – ONS (www.ons.gov.uk)

We are responsible for collecting and publishing statistics related to the economy, population and society at national, regional and local levels. We also conduct the census in England and Wales every ten years.

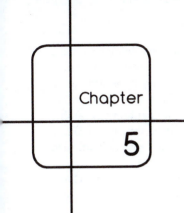

Infection control in settings

Gillian Rowe and Debbie Gee

Chapter aims

After reading this chapter, you will be able to:

1.   understand the importance of good infection control;
2.   identify and apply the legislation, protocols and procedures that govern infection control;
3.   define the core principles that ensure safe, effective work for patients, colleagues, and the environment;
4.   understand how infection control supports the promotion of good health.

Introduction

Good infection prevention (including cleanliness) is essential to ensure that people who use health and social care services receive safe and effective care. Effective prevention and control of infection must be part of everyday practice and be applied consistently by everyone.

(DH, 2015)

The importance of good infection control, antimicrobial stewardship and vaccination has been thrown into sharp relief since the Covid-19 pandemic. Members of the public have had to develop an awareness of infection control and the importance of handwashing. They have also had to learn how to wear a mask in their day-to-day life. Nearly all of us have adapted to incorporating infection control measures at home, at work and while out and about. This chapter will examine the history of public health and infection prevention, Personal Protective Equipment (PPE) and antimicrobial stewardship. We will then consider the chain of infection and sepsis. We will also consider the safe handling of contaminated material and safe food hygiene.

Covid-19 apart, why do we still need to reinforce the principles of infection control? Guest et al. (2020) estimate that 653,000 (2017 figures) patients a year in England acquire a healthcare-associated infection (HAI), of which 22,800 patients died because of their infection (figures for Scotland, Wales and NI not given). Included within those figures are a significant number of NHS employees who acquired a HAI at their workplace. The most common types of healthcare-associated infection are respiratory infections (including pneumonia and infections of the lower respiratory tract; 22.8 per cent), urinary tract infections (17.2 per cent) and surgical site infections (15.7 per cent) (NICE, 2020c). The growth in HAIs can be attributed to invasive procedures and diagnostic tests, mixing of patient populations as hospitals take in from wider catchment areas, and pressure on beds leading to higher levels of in-hospital patient movements.

Pressure for beds can lead to rushed bed cleansing between patients resulting in weaker standards of cleanliness and hygiene, and the growth of antimicrobial resistant organisms. Therefore, infection control is about preventing premature deaths and caring for people in a safe environment and protecting them from avoidable harm. Infection control is a health promoting activity.

History of public health and infection control

The UK has a long history of attempting to control infections. Arguably the greatest public health event was the recognition that sewerage and drinking water should be separated. Cities like London had a patch work approach to dealing with sewerage. The tributary rivers of the Thames such as the Tyburn and the Fleet were open sewers. Night soil men collected buckets of human waste which were dumped in the Thames. During the hot summer of 1858, the smell from the river was so bad that Parliament considered abandoning the city. Called 'the great stink', the city was plagued by cholera, typhus, flies and rats. Parliament rushed through a bill in 18 days to provide the money for a public sewerage scheme which cost £2.4 million (about a £1 billion in current money). Under the Public Health Act 1848, there had been many previous attempts at building sewers in the UK, but the legislation was ineffective, and the government policy was 'laissez faire' (leave well alone). However, the act did set up health boards based on the recommendations made by Edwin Chadwick in his report 'On the sanitary conditions of the labouring population of Great Britain' (1838). The health boards were obliged to report to parliament on sewerage, clean water and infectious diseases. From then on, incremental improvements were made in the prevention and control of disease. The remit was widened to include inadequate housing, poor and adulterated food (poor nutrition), hazardous workplaces and pollution.

Change comes slowly to the medical profession, who are not noted as early adopters of progressive ideas. For instance, Snow's assertion that cholera is waterborne was not accepted until after his death. Semmelweis's (1847) theory that doctors hands carried decaying bacteria between autopsies and pregnant women and thus caused puerperal fever, so physicians should wash their hands, was totally rejected. It was not until the work of Lister in 1870 that handwashing became an accepted practice.

Joseph Lister (1827–1912) and Florence Nightingale (1820–1910) pioneered many of the hospital infection control measures we still use today. Lister, following on from the work of Semmelweis, pioneered antiseptic surgery and promoted the notion of sterile surgery. He also championed the use of carbolic acid (phenol) as an antiseptic to clean wounds. Famously, Nightingale took 38 nurses to the Crimean war in Russia and set up a hospital where she introduced basic infection control measures (handwashing and clean drinking water). Nightingale was credited with reducing the death rate from 42 per cent to 2 per cent.

Antimicrobial resistance and infection prevention

Hand hygiene is an important factor in reducing the spread of healthcare-associated infections (HAIs).

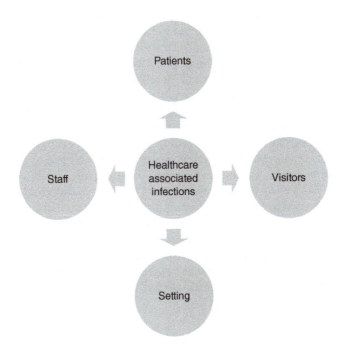

Figure 5.1   HAI infections

Antimicrobial resistance (AMR) is the ability of microorganisms to resist antimicrobial treatments such as antibiotics. The risk of treatment failure and reduced treatment options had led to reduced prescribing of antibiotics to diminish antibiotic resistance. Healthcare-associated infections (previously known as hospital-acquired infections) are infections a patient acquires in a healthcare setting. These impact negatively on those who suffer the pain and distress of the infection, leading to long-term complications and lengthened hospital stays. Methicillin-resistant staphylococcus aureus (MRSA) is a case in point.

Staphylococcus aureus (SA) become resistant to penicillin in the 1940s, shortly after the introduction of the drug. Methicillin was developed in 1959 as a semi-synthetic pharmacokinetic to evade resistance mechanisms to treat penicillin resistant infections. However, by the early 1960s, reports came from the UK and Europe that SA had mutated and become resistant. Methicillin was superseded by oxacillin due to renal complications caused by the drug, so although the drug is no longer in general use, somehow the name stuck. Adverse publicity regarding MRSA deaths in healthcare settings led to a loss of public confidence and staff morale suffered consequently.

MRSA, popularly labelled a 'superbug', became a problem, as it thrives in healthcare settings. It usually colonises the skin and nose, leading to complications and premature death after surgical intervention or treatment for open wounds. It is prevalent in hospitals, prisons and nursing homes, where people with open wounds, invasive devices such as cannula, nasogastric tubes, catheters and weakened immune systems are at greater risk.

The Panton-valentine leucocidin (PVL-MRSA) toxin destroys white blood cells when it colonises an open wound. It can cause necrotising pneumonia, which rapidly destroys lung tissue and is lethal in 75 per cent of cases. PVL-MRSA microbes contain high levels of proteins which make them stickier, therefore easier to adhere to skin and thus spread via contaminated hands.

MRSA has now escaped into the community (community acquired MRSA or CA-MRSA) and has gone on to infect not just humans but livestock (LA-MRSA) also.

Prevention and control rely on effective early detection, so contact precautions need to be put into place to prevent **transmission**. MRSA reveals itself by spots that look like a pimple or acne, but quickly turns into a hard, painful red lump filled with pus or a cluster of pus-filled blisters (boils). Further on in the chapter we will discuss transmission prevention measures.

Other antibiotic resistant organisms include Extended Spectrum Beta-Lactamase (ESBL) and Carbapenemase-producing Enterobacteriaceae (CPE), these are enzymes normally produced by microorganisms in the gut, such as E. coli and Klebsiella. In a healthy person, they are usually harmless, but they can cause infections in the gut and in the bloodstream. These bacteria are spread through direct contact (person to person) or by touching equipment. They are difficult to treat, and PPE should always be worn and handwashing vigilance maintained. Vancomycin-Resistant Enterococcus (VRE) generally affects those who have been taking antibiotics over an extended period of time, or who have had abdominal or chest surgery or have an indwelling catheter. It can lead to meningitis and endocarditis. Usually, patients with VRE are nursed in a private room and the care team should wear PPE to convention. As VRE is spread by direct contact, care should be taken cleansing any equipment and vigilant handwashing is essential.

Other HAIs include Norovirus (winter vomiting), Clostridium difficile, E. coli, klebsiella and gram-negative bacterial infections. These are currently under surveillance by Public Health England.

The NHS produced a standard infection control precautions framework based on the Health and Social Care Act (2008) code of practice on the prevention and control of infections and related guidance. This legislates for compliance with infection prevention and control. All staff must:

1. *Show their understanding by applying the infection prevention and control principles, and maintain competence, skills and knowledge in infection prevention and control by attending education events and/or completing training.*
2. *Communicate the infection prevention and control practices to be carried out by colleagues, those being cared for, relatives and visitors, without breaching confidentiality.*
3. *Have up-to-date occupational immunisations, health checks and clearance requirements.*
4. *Report to line managers and document any deficits in knowledge, resources, equipment and facilities or incidents that may result in transmitting infection including near misses, for instance PPE failures.*
5. *Not provide care while at risk of transmitting infectious agents to others, if in doubt, they must consult their line manager, occupational health department, infection prevention and control team (IPCT) or health protection team (HPT).*

(nhsengland.org, 2019)

Standard infection control precautions

The NHS has various directives regarding infection control and each trust and clinical setting will have their own policies in effect. It is recommended that settings adopt a 'bare below the elbow' approach with attention on the hands, no stoned rings (plain bands), no false nails or nail extensions and preferably no wrist watches, a nurse's fob watch being ideal.

Hand hygiene

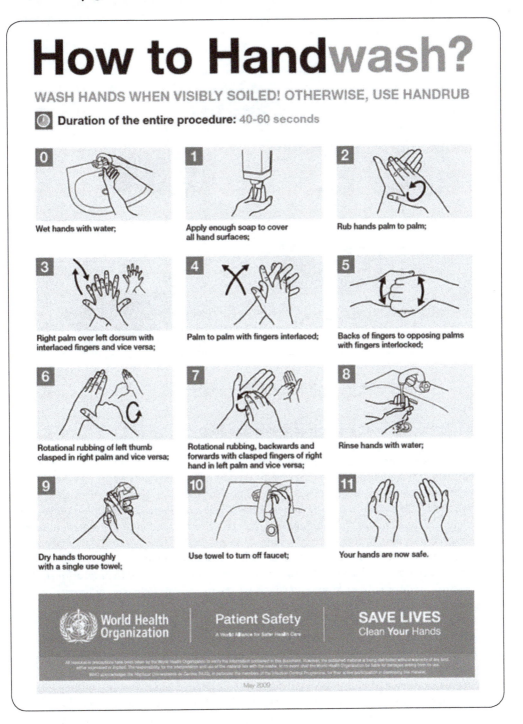

How to Handwash?

WASH HANDS WHEN VISIBLY SOILED! OTHERWISE, USE HANDRUB

Duration of the entire procedure: 40-60 seconds

0 Wet hands with water;

1 Apply enough soap to cover all hand surfaces;

2 Rub hands palm to palm;

3 Right palm over left dorsum with interlaced fingers and vice versa;

4 Palm to palm with fingers interlaced;

5 Backs of fingers to opposing palms with fingers interlocked;

6 Rotational rubbing of left thumb clasped in right palm and vice versa;

7 Rotational rubbing, backwards and forwards with clasped fingers of right hand in left palm and vice versa;

8 Rinse hands with water;

9 Dry hands thoroughly with a single use towel;

10 Use towel to turn off faucet;

11 Your hands are now safe.

World Health Organization | Patient Safety
A World Alliance for Safer Health Care | SAVE LIVES Clean Your Hands

May 2009

Figure 5.2 WHO handwashing guide

The World Health Organization (WHO, 2021a) maintain that hands are the main pathways of germ transmission during healthcare. Examine the image of the WHO handwashing guide (Figure 5.2) in order to ensure your hand-washing technique is correct and no areas of your hands are unwashed, ensure you remove any rings first. The best handwashing uses soap and hot water and hands dried using disposable paper towels. Gels with 70+ per cent alcohol should be used as a backup, rather than replacing handwashing.

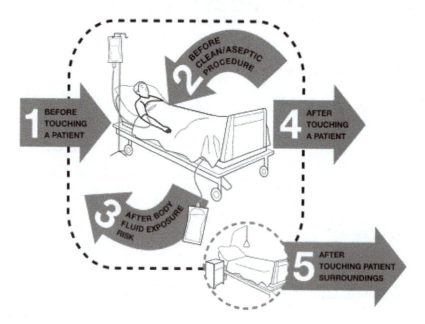

Figure 5.3   Five moments for hand hygiene (WHO, 2021a)

WHO (2021b) state that handwashing should take place:

1.   *Before patient contact, including arrival on duty.*
2.   *After using toilet facilities.*
3.   *Before undertaking an aseptic task, e.g., dressings, intravenous fluid administration.*
4.   *After body fluid exposure risk, including after gloves are removed. Remember gloves may become damaged in use (the damage may be visible or microscopic) therefore hands may also be contaminated accidentally when gloves are being removed and the environment inside the glove may promote microbial growth on the user's hands.*
5.   *Handwashing after taking off gloves may also remove particles of the material that the gloves are made of, such as latex, and so reduce the risk of developing an allergy.*
6.   *After patient contact, such as moving and handling.*
7.   *After contact with patient surroundings, such as the bed and bedding.*
8.   *Before and after any intervention involving body fluid exposure risk, irrespective of whether gloves are worn or not. Gloves do not replace the need for handwashing.*

Covid-19 respiratory and cough prevention offers enhanced handwashing advice such as handwashing after you blow your nose, sneeze, cough and before you handle or eat food. WHO (2021b) promote water, sanitation and hygiene (WASH) practices and recommend frequent and proper handwashing to prevent infection transmission. The main means of Covid-19 transmission is by respiratory droplets and aerosols when people talk, cough and sneeze, which can be inhaled by people close by. WHO recommend hygiene stations should be available at all points of care and in areas where PPE is put on or taken off (donning and doffing). Hand hygiene should also be available to visitors such as family and friends.

There are two types of microorganisms that carry the risk of infection and contamination.

1. Transient: found on skin surface, readily acquired from contact with other body sites, people and the environment, easily transferred to others.
2. Resident microorganisms: normal skin flora found in deeper skin layers, hair follicles and sweat glands, more difficult to remove than transient microorganisms.

Extra protection once hands have been washed would be advocated by the infection control team (ICT) during outbreaks of infection. Antiseptic solutions include chlorhexidine gluconate, povidone iodine, and alcohol hand rub (70+ per cent). There is a risk from these products such as skin irritation, accidental eye splashes, ingestion, and fire hazard (alcohol hand rub).

Promoting your own health

Skin protection is essential as damaged skin is a portal for infection. Facial personal protective equipment (PPE) worn for extended periods of time can cause facial skin damage due to pressure effects, so your mask should be removed as often as possible. Barrier cream can be applied, and the skin gently massaged, although you must do this 30 minutes before donning a fitted respirator mask. A skin barrier film or liquid skin protectant could be applied on the bridge of your nose, your cheekbones and behind your ears. Check your hands regularly for signs of redness and abrasion and use a good quality hand moisturiser as often as possible.

Personal protective equipment (PPE)

Employers have duties concerning PPE. The Personal Protective Equipment at Work Regulations (1992) Regulation 4 states 'personal protective equipment' means all equipment (including clothing affording protection against the weather) which is intended to be worn or held by a person at work and which protects him against one or more risks to his health or safety. The primary uses of personal protective equipment are to protect staff and patients in NHS and community settings. NICE (2014, 2017) state that 'The decision to use or wear personal protective equipment must be based upon an assessment of the level of risk associated with a specific patient care activity or intervention and take account of current health and safety legislation'. Each setting and care provider will have protocols and policies that determine under what circumstance PPE is to be worn. It is for you to familiarise yourself with your settings' guidelines. Each employer must provide, at no cost to you, PPE to ensure your safety, your patient's safety and to reduce the transmission of microorganisms which could cause healthcare associated infections (HAIs). Other legislation includes the Health and Safety at Work Act (1974), the Control of Substances Hazardous to Health Regulations (2002) and the Management of Health and Safety at Work Regulations (1999).

Most PPE is single use only and disposable. Single-use equipment such as gowns or coveralls should never be washed, as it removes the protective elements. Some masks, respirators and hoods are reusable, and these are discussed further in the chapter.

Gloves: used for invasive procedures, contact with sterile sites and non-intact skin or mucous membranes, as well as all activities with risk of exposure to blood, body fluids, secretions and excretions, and when handling sharp or contaminated instruments (more on sharps further in the chapter). Gloves should not be worn unnecessarily as their prolonged and indiscriminate use may cause adverse reactions and skin sensitivity. Figure 5.4 shows you the WHO glove pyramid, which indicates what kind of glove should be worn and when. Gloves should be strictly single use only and should be disposed of to convention. Be mindful how you remove your gloves, contamination can happen, so ensure you wash your hands carefully after removing gloves.

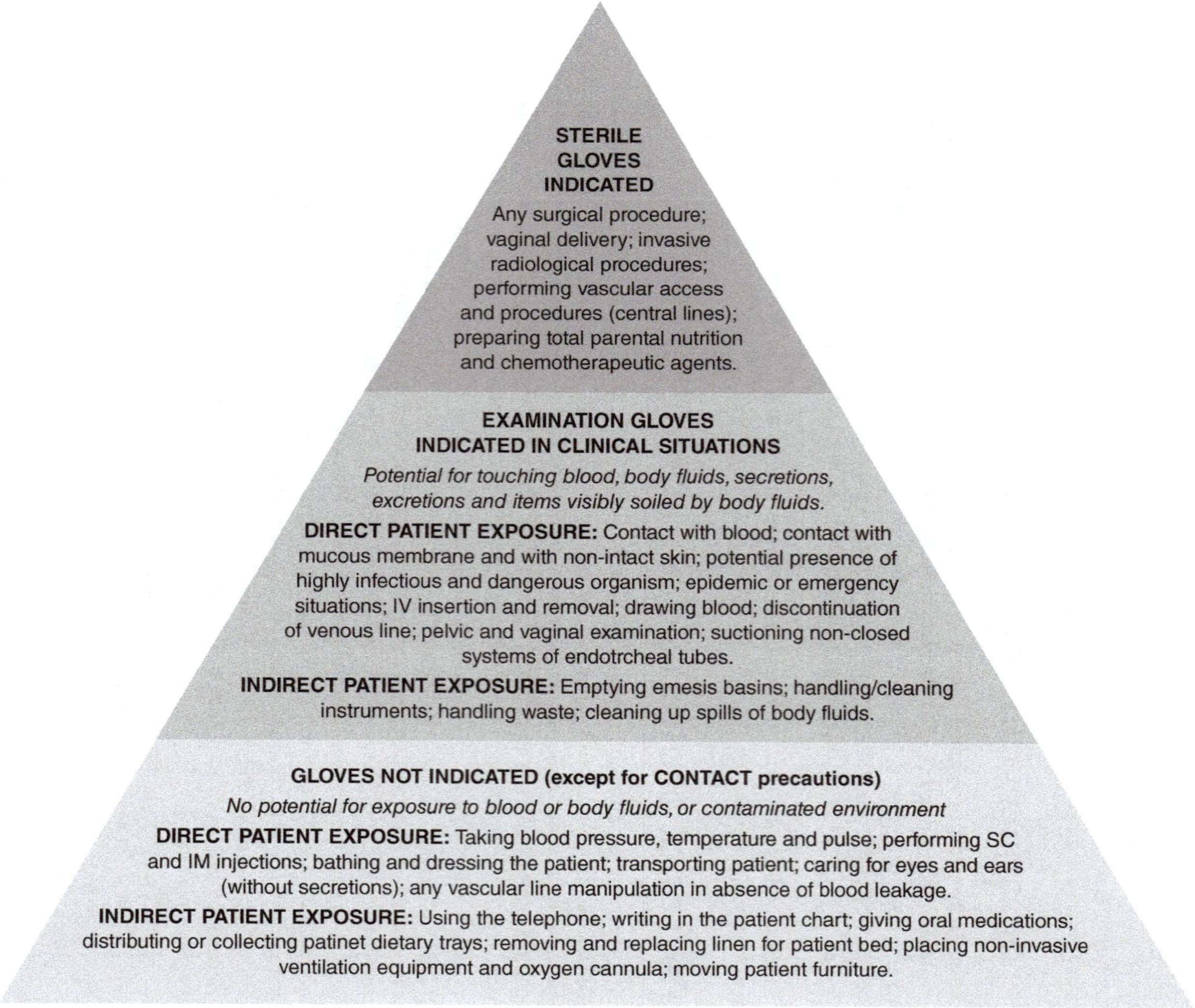

STERILE GLOVES INDICATED

Any surgical procedure; vaginal delivery; invasive radiological procedures; performing vascular access and procedures (central lines); preparing total parental nutrition and chemotherapeutic agents.

EXAMINATION GLOVES INDICATED IN CLINICAL SITUATIONS

Potential for touching blood, body fluids, secretions, excretions and items visibly soiled by body fluids.

DIRECT PATIENT EXPOSURE: Contact with blood; contact with mucous membrane and with non-intact skin; potential presence of highly infectious and dangerous organism; epidemic or emergency situations; IV insertion and removal; drawing blood; discontinuation of venous line; pelvic and vaginal examination; suctioning non-closed systems of endotrcheal tubes.

INDIRECT PATIENT EXPOSURE: Emptying emesis basins; handling/cleaning instruments; handling waste; cleaning up spills of body fluids.

GLOVES NOT INDICATED (except for CONTACT precautions)

No potential for exposure to blood or body fluids, or contaminated environment

DIRECT PATIENT EXPOSURE: Taking blood pressure, temperature and pulse; performing SC and IM injections; bathing and dressing the patient; transporting patient; caring for eyes and ears (without secretions); any vascular line manipulation in absence of blood leakage.

INDIRECT PATIENT EXPOSURE: Using the telephone; writing in the patient chart; giving oral medications; distributing or collecting patinet dietary trays; removing and replacing linen for patient bed; placing non-invasive ventilation equipment and oxygen cannula; moving patient furniture.

Figure 5.4 WHO glove pyramid

Aprons: used when in close contact with patients, materials or equipment where clothing may be contaminated with pathogenic microorganisms or blood, body fluids, secretions or excretions (excluding perspiration). Aprons have a demonstrable role in prevention of cross infection, so aprons should be changed when moving between patients and at the end of an activity. Apron removal should be to convention, and they should be disposed of according to your setting's protocols.

Full-body fluid-repellent gowns or coveralls: used when there is a risk of extensive splashing onto your skin or clothing of blood, body fluids, secretions or excretions may occur. These gowns should always be worn in Covid-19 'hot' areas due to risk of droplet/aerosol contamination.

Eye protection: should be worn when there is a risk of blood, body fluids, secretions or excretions splashing into the face and eyes. Face visors are a type of face shield made from a transparent material and can be held in place by a band that goes around the head, or by sliding the visor onto glasses.

Face masks: Under normal circumstances, surgical face masks are only worn when undertaking procedures that carry a risk of contamination. However, Covid-19 pandemic instructions (2021) are that all healthcare care staff, in any setting, should wear surgical masks for the duration of their shift. Clear face masks should be available for those who work with patients who lip read or who use facial expressions as a primary form of communication.

Surgical face masks are loose fitting, cover the nose and mouth, and are designed to protect the patient from bacteria shed in liquid droplets and aerosols coming from your nose and mouth. They are single use and are generally changed every two hours, and they are disposed of in clinical waste bags. They are classified as Class 1 Medical Devices under the Medical Devices Directive (93/42/EEC).

Respiratory masks must meet the more rigorous European safety standard EN149, the standard being FFP1, 2(II), 3 (IIR), the differences between the masks lies within their bacterial filtration efficiency. All filter a differing percentage of particles. Type I face masks have a bacterial filtration efficiency of >=95 per cent, whereas Type II and Type IIR face masks have a bacterial filtration efficiency of >=98 per cent. Type IIR are splash resistant and should be used in Covid-19 'hot' areas. They can be valved or non-valved and can be single use or reusable. Valved masks make exhaling easier and so are a little more comfortable than non-valved. Respirator masks are usually used during aerosol-generating procedures (AGP). These masks are considered the safer option in Covid-19 wards.

Reusable respiratory protective equipment (RRPE) must be correctly sized and fitted (the fit test) and used when nursing patients with airborne respiratory infections. Personal respiratory protection is required in certain respiratory diseases, e.g., Covid-19, HIV-related and multiple drug-resistant tuberculosis. Reusable respirators should never be shared, and yours should be labelled and stored in a manner that reduces risk of transmission.

Fit test

There are two types of fit tests: Qualitative and quantitative fit.

Qualitative fit testing is a pass–fail test that uses the sense of taste or smell and the user's reaction to an irritant in order to detect leakage into the respirator's face piece.

Quantitative fit testing uses a machine to measure the actual amount of leakage into the face piece.

The qualitative fit test requires you to check if the mask has a tight seal to your skin, a bitter (or sweet) tasting agent is sprayed on the mask, and if you detect it, the mask has failed the test. The fit test should be undertaken by someone assessed as competent to undertake fit tests. This is to ensure that the respiratory protective equipment will protect you. If you gain or lose weight, you may need a different type of FFP mask. A fit check should be undertaken each time a new mask is put on (donned) and you should be trained on how to do the fit check. The HSE has a training video to watch to ensure your knowledge is correct and up to date. The web address is given at the end of this chapter in the useful websites section. The HSE poster (Figure 5.5) shows you how to correctly fit the respirator. Reusable masks should be cleaned to convention, and you should be trained in the correct cleaning methods.

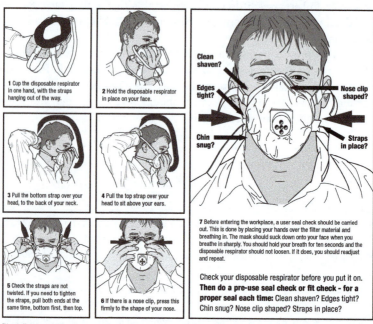

Figure 5.5   Using disposable respirators

If you cannot wear a respirator, you could be offered a non-disposable powered hood, as these do not require a fit test. Powered hoods should be cleaned with a recommended disinfectant wipe, inside and out, and left to air dry. If it has a nebuliser, this should be removed and immersed in a disinfectant liquid, along with any tubing, then left to air dry. Attention should be paid to the cleaning process, as quite often this piece of PPE is shared due to shortages.

Antimicrobial stewardship

In order to understand what an antimicrobial is, we need to understand what microbes are. These are microscopic single-celled living things that are categorised into groups of microorganisms: bacteria, fungi (yeasts and molds), protozoa and algae. While viruses and prions are microscopic, they are not classed as living things. The human body is colonised by millions of microorganisms collectively known as the human microbiota. They are found on the skin, and all the orifices (nose, mouth, ears, penis, vargina and urethra). Bacteria are larger than viruses and are capable of reproducing on their own. Viruses (see Figure 5.7) cannot reproduce on their own. Instead, they reproduce by infecting a host and using the host's DNA replication systems to make copies of itself.

You have on average about 100,000 bacteria on every square centimetre of your skin. These dine on the ten billion flakes of skin that you shed every day, plus all the oils and minerals that you secrete. There are trillions more inside your gut, they reproduce in less than ten minutes, so in 24 hours one can become 280,000 billion. Bacteria come in three basic shapes: rod-shaped (bacilli), spherical (cocci) or helical (spirilla) (see Figure 5.6 for various types of bacteria). Bacteria are also classified as gram-positive or gram-negative. Gram-positive bacteria have a thick cell wall while gram-negative bacteria do not.

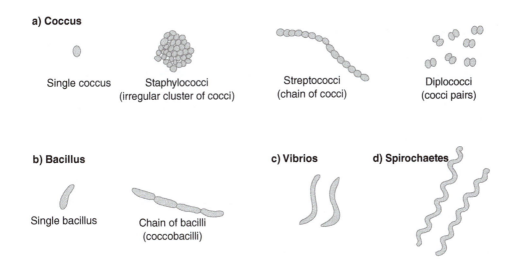

a) Coccus

Single coccus Staphylococci (irregular cluster of cocci) Streptococci (chain of cocci) Diplococci (cocci pairs)

b) Bacillus **c) Vibrios** **d) Spirochaetes**

Single bacillus Chain of bacilli (coccobacilli)

Figure 5.6 Bacteria

Some bacteria are essential for body functioning. These are called commensals as they co-exist peacefully with us, supporting digestion, production and synthesis of vitamins B and K, promoting the development of the immune system and detoxifying harmful chemicals.

Some bacteria and yeasts are harmless until the environment is disturbed. An example of this is Candida Albicans, which can cause candidiasis, better known as thrush (oral, vaginal and penile). Usually mild and irritating, Candida can become invasive via the vascular system and infect the brain or organs. This is problematic for those with compromised immune systems.

Candida Auris is an emerging fungus that presents a serious global health threat as it is multi-resistant to all classes of antifungals.

Harmful strains of bacteria can infect any part of the body. See Table 5.1 for examples of different common bacterial infections and the ailments they cause.

Table 5.1 Examples of bacterial infections

Staphylococcus	Boils, cellulitis, Bacteraemia, food poisoning, endocarditis, Toxic shock syndrome, pneumonia
Streptococcus	Pneumonia, endocarditis, sepsis, impetigo, throat infections (strep throat)
Campylobacter jejuni	Diarrhoea cramp, fever
Clostridium botulinum (botulism)	Diarrhoea, produces neurotoxins
Clostridium difficile (C.dif.)	Diarrhoea, colitis, sepsis
Escherichia coli (E. coli)	Diarrhoea cramp fever
Listeria monocytogenes	Diarrhoea cramp fever
Chlamydia	Pelvic inflammatory disease, infertility
Bacterial meningitis	Inflammation of the meninges (lining of the brain)
Tuberculosis	Respiratory tract infection

Antibiotic resistance

Antibiotic resistance occurs when bacteria are no longer sensitive to a medication that should eliminate an infection. This dangerous situation has occurred for several reasons:

1. Over-prescription of antibiotics: Also, in some countries, antibiotics are available over the counter.
2. Patients not finishing the entire antibiotic course: People stopped taking the medication when they felt better or because it upset their stomachs. This allowed live bacteria the opportunity to mutate so that the drug became ineffective.
3. Overuse of antibiotics in livestock and fish farming: Antibiotics were given to livestock as a prophylactic to prevent disease, but it was found they encouraged growth in animals and fish, so antibiotics were routinely added to food.
4. Undercooked meat and raw fish allowed pathogenic-resistant organisms into the food chain, and they may act as **reservoirs** for resistant bacteria.
5. Poor infection control in healthcare settings: larger hospitals are taking patients from wider geographic areas bringing more patients into contact who then spread pathogens into their own community. Rapid churn of patients and demand for beds means that time spent cleaning the environment is skimped allowing pathogenic spread.
6. Lack of new antibiotic drugs coming to market: Drug companies feel the returns for developing new antibiotics are not worth the investment, this is because most governments around the world cap the price they will pay for drugs.

Viruses are small particles of genetic material (either DNA or RNA) that are surrounded by a protein coat. Some viruses also have a fatty envelope covering. Common viral infections include influenza, measles, mumps and rubella, HIV/AIDs, hepatitis (B and C), croup, noro- and rotor virus and Covid-19. Viruses are also implicated in the development of cancer. Some viruses have the ability to go dormant (or quiescent) and then reactivate after a trigger. The herpes simplex virus can reactivate in reaction to stress, fever, menstruation and exposure to sunlight.

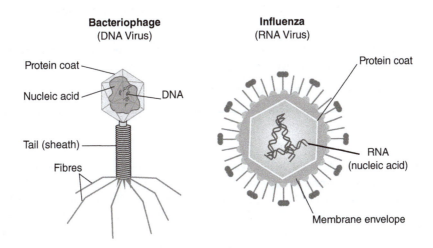

Figure 5.7   A virus

As viruses are not entirely alive, they are difficult to destroy. The search for drugs that could kill viruses came out of the HIV/AIDs **epidemic**. HIV/AIDs is a zoonotic virus that moved from the monkey population to humans in the Democratic Republic of Congo. The disease spread slowly during the 1970s but then it entered the American gay population, and it was originally called a gay plague. By 1983, the novel disease was given the name of 'Acquired Immune Deficiency syndrome'. AIDs, however, is not contagious. It was later found that the retrovirus human immunodeficiency virus (HIV) was the causative of AIDs. While a person who has AIDS has HIV, not every person with HIV will develop AIDS.

Huge sums of money and many institutions have been engaged in developing antiretroviral drugs and vaccines. While a cure for HIV has yet to be found, drugs are slowing down the effects of the disease. With the challenge of finding drugs to combat SARs-CoV-2, antiretrovirals are being repurposed. Research efforts are building on previous research on severe acute respiratory syndrome (SARS) and Middle East respiratory syndrome (MERS), which also are caused by coronaviruses. Hopefully, bringing these research capabilities together will bridge knowledge gaps and lead to a positive outcome.

NICE (2015, 2020) define antimicrobial stewardship (AMS) as 'an organisational or healthcare-system-wide approach to promoting and monitoring judicious use of antimicrobials to preserve their future effectiveness'. According to Resman (2020), 'work in antimicrobial stewardship is complex and includes not only aspects of infectious disease and microbiology, but also of epidemiology, genetics, behavioural psychology, systems science, economics and ethics'. It is well-established that increased use of antibiotics has led to increased antibiotic resistance. Agricultural use of antibiotics has led to both food and the environment being contaminated with antibiotic residues. Antibiotic overuse and misuse through prescribing practice has increased microorganisms resistant to antibiotics in both populations and individuals. Quite often, patients will ask for antibiotics when they are not needed but do not understand why their request has been refused. Read Activity 5.1 and consider your responses to Valerie.

Activity 5.1   Critical thinking

Valerie complains to you that her GP will no longer prescribe antibiotics for a sore throat. She then says she does not think the antibiotics work anyway and she doesn't always complete the course as they upset her stomach.

From the information Valerie has given you, surmise what is likely causing her upset stomach and what advice would you give her to protect herself in future.

Compare your answer with the answer given at the end of the chapter.

What Valerie does not understand is that taking unnecessary antibiotics can lead to unwanted side effects. Antibiotics are not very specific and can kill helpful bacteria leaving the body open to opportunistic invasive bacteria and yeast infections such as Clostridium Difficile (C. dif.) and thrush. Research by Palleja et al. (2018) showed that a diverse gut microbiota is considered to promote health, but that poor microbiotic diversity has a relationship with chronic ailments such as obesity, diabetes, asthma and alimentary inflammatory disorders. Their research also showed that the gut can take up to six months to recover from antibiotic therapy and that that colonisation by non-desirable bacteria occurs.

Antibiotic reaction

According to Blumenthal et al. (2019), antibiotics are the commonest cause of life-threatening immune-mediated drug reactions. However, they go to state that very few patient-reported allergies are thoroughly investigated. Patients who report allergies to antibiotics frequently cannot remember which antibiotic provoked a reaction, so they often cite an allergy to penicillin. This reduces their access to therapeutic intervention. Antibiotic reactions range from nausea, bloating, diarrhoea, lip swelling, urticaria, wheezing, tightness around the throat and anaphylaxis (difficulty breathing and collapse). Quite often, an antihistamine is sufficient to mediate the symptoms, however, Fluoroquinolone can provoke muscle and joint pain, tingling and numbness, which are considered serious side effects. Accurate documentation is essential when a patient reports side effects. You should listen to their concerns and if the patient experiences any serious symptoms, you should escalate to the clinical team.

The chain of infection

As you can see, the chain of infection is an interlocking sequence of events that allow infection to be spread. If the chain is broken at any point, the opportunity for contagion is reduced.

1. The infectious agent: these are the pathogens that cause diseases, these can be bacteria, virus, fungi or parasites.
2. The reservoir: this is the host that allows the pathogen to reproduce. Humans, animals, insects, fish, water and the environment are all possible hosts.
3. The portal of exit: this is the route the agent takes to leaves the host, an example might be sneezing, coughing, blood or faeces.
4. Mode of transmission: this could be direct contact with the agent (insect bite) indirect contact by airborne transmission, ingestion, or fomites (objects likely to be contaminated, e.g., bedding, equipment)

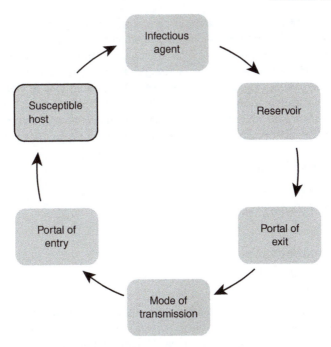

Figure 5.8 Chain of infection

5. Portal of entry: this could be absorption into a mucus membrane, ingestion via the GI tract, inhalation into the respiratory tract, broken skin such as injury, injection, small cut, abrasion. Clinical procedure such as catheterisation.
6. Susceptible host: someone who is immunocompromised, post-surgery, open wounds, cardiopulmonary disease, predisposing factors.

Breaking the chain:

1. The infectious agent: early identification of the causative agent means correct and effective treatment.
2. The reservoir: environmental sanitation (clean water, clean air) healthy uncontaminated food, clean working environment.
3. The portal of exit: control of excretions, proper handwashing, effective waste disposal, wearing PPE.
4. Mode of transmission: food handling training, effective surface cleaning, wearing PPE for disposal of contaminated materials, good laundry care (washing at 70° temperature), control of airflow in settings.
5. Portal of entry: handwashing, wearing PPE, aseptic technique for wound dressing, catheter care, safe infection control.
6. Susceptible host: separate patients (elderly, children, immunocompromised) from those with known infections. For patients with open wounds, use appropriate wound care protocols, vaccinations, maintain sanitation.

Sepsis

Sepsis is an extreme reaction to infection and is a life-threatening emergency, defined by organ dysfunction and a dysregulated immune response. Those most at risk of sepsis are the young, elderly, the immunocompromised and those with existing chronic ailments. Sepsis can be life changing, with 40 per cent of patients suffering from lifelong associated ailments and susceptibility to infection. Many sepsis survivors also suffer cognitive decline and poor mental health (PTSD). Sepsis can be caused by a bacterial, viral or fungal infection, although generally the cause is bacterial. Sepsis can progress from sepsis to severe sepsis (organ dysfunction) to septic shock (sustained reduction in arterial blood pressure leading to lack of oxygen in the tissues) quite rapidly. If you suspect sepsis, you must swiftly escalate your concerns to the clinical team and document events.

The Sepsis Trust (sepsisturst.org) define the signs and symptoms using sepsis as an acronym:

Slurred speech or confusion

Extreme shivering or muscle pain

Passing no urine (in a day)

Severe breathlessness

It feels like you're going to die

Skin mottled or discoloured

The symptoms for children are: rapid respirations; convulsions; cyanosed (blue) mottled skin; a rash that does not fade when pressed (the glass test); lethargic and difficult to rouse; maybe floppy; feels cold to the touch; temperature above 38 degrees; not passed urine for 12 hours.

In the UK, the National Early Warning Score (NEWS2) is a diagnostic track and trigger for the deteriorating patient. Any patient who scores three and above is at risk of sepsis. This is in line with the NICE quality statement (NICE, 2020c). Elderly patients with pneumonia or a urinary tract infection account for 70 per cent of sepsis and so these patients should be closely monitored, any changes documented and concerns escalated to the medical team.

Isolation nursing

Sometimes, patients need to be cared for in isolation, called source isolation, because the patient is the source of infection. During the time of Covid-19, cohort isolation was used. Wards became Covid-19 wards, as there were too many patients with Covid-19 and not enough single rooms. Preferably, isolated patients should be nursed by designated staff who are not caring for other patients. The patient should be risk assessed, which considers the source of infection, route of transmission and susceptibility of others.

Precautions include:

- hand hygiene;
- wearing PPE, and safe disposal;
- safe removal of contaminated waste;
- safe removal of bed linen;
- decontamination of reusable equipment.

When single rooms are used, ventilation systems can be utilised to create negative pressure in the isolation room (i.e., the pressure in the room is less than surrounding areas). The aim of this is to prevent air from the room escaping into other areas of the ward. Air from the room is extracted outside of the building. If possible, the use of fans should be avoided to prevent infection transmission. You should understand that patients in isolation will become bored and lonely. If they become anxious, they are less likely to recover well. Activity 5.2 will help you to reflect on what it feels like to be scared and on your own. Patients should be regularly assessed so that they do not stay in isolation longer than they need to. Any visitors should be shown how to wear protective equipment so that they do not become infected.

Activity 5.2   Reflection

Reflect on what it might be like to be cared for in isolation and what you would want from healthcare staff in these circumstances. Think about the things you could do to support a patient in isolation.

A model answer is given at the end of the chapter.

Many people in hospital, but especially those in isolation, become frustrated that their routines have been disrupted, such as being able to get a drink or snack when they want one. Patients' relatives should be encouraged to bring items in for the patient to ease their discomfort.

Safe handling of contaminated material

Laundry

There are three types of contaminated laundry:

1. soiled: used linen generally;
2. fouled: urine, mucus, vomit, faeces, diarrhoea, blood (and blood in vomit);
3. infected: diarrhoea caused by an infectious agent, pus, leakage from wounds, blood from an infectious patient.

Safe handling requires PPE (apron and gloves), depending on the setting and conventions. Many settings use soluble alginate bags, which are bags that dissolve in a hot wash. Alginate bags that are used in a domestic washing machine should have 'seam burst' as they do not fully dissolve in lower domestic machine temperatures and can clog the machine.

All soluble bags must be placed directly into the washing machine to minimise contact, and prevent transmission of infection to laundry staff, or contamination of the environment. Soluble bags are then placed into a red linen bag.

Use a linen skip with an appropriately coloured bag(s) and used linen must always be bagged at the bedside. Used linen should not be placed on the floor or furniture, also it should never be carried through the ward or corridors to the sluice/dirty utility room or laundry. Without shaking the linen, you should check that foreign objects have not been forgotten (syringes, equipment, dressings, etc.) before it goes into the linen bag. Finally, laundry bags must never be more than two-thirds full, so that they can be tied properly. Always carry bags by the neck. Do not hold them against your body and do not throw them, as the bags might burst, spilling the contents.

Used laundry bags should be safely stored until collection, or in non-NHS settings, to company convention.

Some settings encourage residents to do their own laundry, either as a therapeutic activity or to encourage autonomy. This is a good opportunity for you to teach the principles of infection control health education, and to ensure other residents are not exposed to an infection risk.

Waste management and decontamination of reusable equipment

Waste can be classified as clinical, hazardous, offensive and waste. Each category is governed by different legislation and statutory instruments. The main legislation is the Health and Safety at Work Act (1974), the Control of Substances Hazardous to Health Regulations (2002), the Environmental

Protection Act (1990), and the Hazardous Waste Regulations (2005), each of these acts have various amendments, and each setting will have protocols and procedures for implementing them. You should find where your employer keeps this information and ensure that you have read and understood it. Breaking these laws can have serious consequences for you, your registration and for your patients. You should have been given waste management training by your employer and instructed as to waste protocols and the risks associated with waste management.

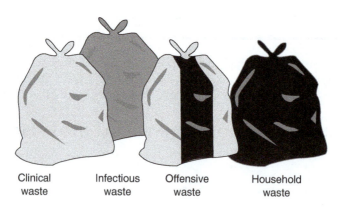

| Clinical waste | Infectious waste | Offensive waste | Household waste |

Figure 5.9   Waste bags

Clinical and hazardous waste comprises anything infectious, chemical hazards and waste drug containers (such as used infusion giving sets, empty infusion bags) which contain active pharmacological materials hazardous to the environment. Clinical waste should be contained in a yellow waste bag, and infectious waste in an orange bag and sent for incineration.

Unused medications and any prescribed lotions and creams should be returned to the pharmacy for safe disposal. Except cytostatic/cytotoxic medicines, which should be placed in identified rigid and sealable containers and sent for incineration.

Offensive waste is non-hazardous hygiene waste, such as used paper hand wipes, and is placed in black and yellow bags for collection and disposal by approved methods. Confidential waste should be placed in identifiable waste containers (usually blue bags) for licenced confidential waste disposal agents.

All waste bags should be tagged or labelled with the name of the generating department, ward or setting so that it can be identified in the event of mishap.

Sharps and needle stick injuries

Disposal of needles and other sharp instruments is governed by the Health and Safety (Sharp Instruments in Healthcare) Regulations (2013). The Care Quality Commission (CQC) state that employers must meet essential standards of quality and safety in keeping patients and staff safe. Employers should have a safer sharps policy where possible. This means using needles safety engineered protection such as a shield or cover that slides or pivots to cover the needle after use.

Regulation 5(1)(c) considers that injuries can occur after a needle has been used if the healthcare worker holds the needle in one hand and attempts to place a cap on the needle with the other hand (so-called two-handed recapping) (hse.gov.uk, 2019). Therefore, needles should never be re-sheathed, but disposed of in a yellow sharps box at the point of use. Other sharps such as lancets, cannulas and suturing needles should also be disposed of in a portable sharps box and not passed hand to hand for disposal.

Needle stick injuries resulting from exposure-prone procedures carry the risk of hepatitis B virus (HBV), hepatitis C virus (HCV) and human immunodeficiency virus (HIV). Although rare, healthcare workers have been infected, with life-changing effects.

Decontamination

There are three types of decontamination, depending on the item being cleansed and the level of hygiene required.

- cleaning: removal of dirt and other physical contamination and some microorganisms;
- disinfection: reduction in numbers of microorganisms but not bacterial spores;
- sterilisation: destruction or removal of all microorganisms including bacterial spores.

Decontamination of communal equipment such as commodes and hoists should be undertaken after each use, using appropriate cleaning fluids and wipes. Your employer will have 'Cleaning and Disinfection' or 'Decontamination' policies which identify the correct methods for decontaminating equipment. Some settings use 'I am clean' tape or cleaning sheets that require a signature to confirm cleaning has taken place. A visible inspection should also be undertaken and if any part of the equipment is found to be faulty then it should not be used. A notice should be put on the equipment, and the repair escalated to the maintenance team.

Cleaning up spills should take place to NHS cleaning standards, and cleaning protocols should include responsibility for cleaning, frequency of cleaning and method of environment decontamination (nhs.uk, 2019). All spillages of blood, body fluids and excreta must be regarded as potentially hazardous and cleared immediately by appropriately trained staff.

Infectious agents on flat surfaces can be cleaned with packs such as 'Clinell™' wipe packs and walls should be decontaminated using such products as 'Actichlor Plus™'. You should remember that chlorine-based products (including bleach) should not be used to clean up urine or vomit. Chlorine and the acid in urine and vomit combined release poisonous chlorine gas.

Protecting yourself

You need to protect yourself from occupational exposure, such as percutaneous injury, exposure of non-intact skin, e.g., cuts, eczema and exposure of your mucous membranes including your eyes. If you do cut or stick yourself, immediately wash the wound or non-intact skin thoroughly with soap and water (do not scrub), gently encourage bleeding of puncture wounds (do not suck) and apply a waterproof dressing. Use copious amount of water to wash your eyes, if affected. It is then essential that you report the incident to your line manager and complete an incident form. You should then attend Occupational Health (or A&E if out of hours).

Food hygiene

Nursing associates do not usually hold a food hygiene certificate unless your role requires you to support food preparation with your clients. However, you do have an important role to play in maintaining standards of food hygiene, this work is covered by the Food Safety Act (1990) and the Food Hygiene (England) Regulations (2006). Hospital and care setting patients are more vulnerable than healthy people to microbiological and nutritional risks.

Catering is often contracted out to private providers, and snack provision provided by a league of friends, however, they are expected to adhere to Hazard Analysis Critical Control Point (HACCP) principles. Food is categorised as low and high risk, low-risk foods are things such as bread, biscuits and cereals. High-risk foods are ready-to-eat foods which support the growth of microorganisms, such as cooked meat and fish, dairy products, baby foods and enteral feeding products.

The infection control team handle food complaints or allegations of food poisoning arising from food/drink provided by trusts and primary care teams. If you give out meals or hot drinks and snacks to patients, you will be classified as a food handler and you will be expected to know the basic principles for handling food. These are based on the NHS food hygiene policy.

- Wash your hands before handling food or kitchen/serving equipment.
- Wash your hands after using the toilet, after sneezing, coughing, or using a handkerchief, or after touching your ears, nose, mouth or hair.
- Avoid unnecessary handling of food.
- Keep all equipment and surfaces clean.
- Follow any food safety instructions on food packaging or ask your line manager.
- Tell your line manager if you see something wrong.
- Patients and visitors are not permitted to use ward kitchens.
- Kitchens in other settings must be secure to ensure that pets, strays, wild animals and birds cannot enter the area.
- Cleaning chemicals and disinfectants must not be stored in areas where food is handled.

You should not handle food if you have any open wounds on your hands, even if they are covered with a waterproof dressing. You should not attend work if you have had a bout of vomiting and diarrhoea until you have been clear of symptoms for 48 hours.

Activity 5.3   Work-based learning

You are working in a residential care setting for young people with a learning disability. It is 2pm in the afternoon and visitors have arrived for Ricky Woodman. His father hands you a carrier bag within which are several plastic food containers. He tells you this is for his son's tea; it is from Ricky's favourite Indian takeaway and it is chicken tikka masala and rice. Mr Woodman asks you to warm it up for his son at teatime.

How would you ensure the food provided by Mr Woodman for his son is hygienic and fit to safely be consumed?

Compare your answers with the answer at the end of the chapter.

Chapter summary

This chapter has introduced you to the theories, legislation and practice of infection control. You will have learned how to promote safe working practice for yourself, your colleagues and your patients. The key takeaways from this chapter are that infection control works within a framework of legislation, protocols and procedures. It is important that you keep yourself up to date when changes are made. When you go to a new placement or employment, you need to understand local policies and how they are implemented. Talk to your mentor or supervisor so that you feel confident in your work.

Activities: Brief outline answers

Activity 5.1 Critical thinking (page 96)

The broad-spectrum antibiotics her GP prescribes could be causing her upset stomach, due to them killing the helpful bacteria and leading to abdominal pain, bloating and diarrhoea. You explain the importance of completing any course of antibiotics, that by stopping taking the antibiotic, some of the bacteria could still be active and this could allow the bacteria to mutate and then the antibiotic would be useless. This is an opportunity to discuss why Valerie is suffering sore throats and to offer advice, self-management strategies and homely remedies (over-the-counter throat pastilles, gargles, paracetamol, when needed, and fluids).

Activity 5.2 Reflection (page 99)

Disconnection from the outside world and being away from families and friends can lead to anxiety related to the uncertainties of the situation. Some fear stigmatisation, as they have been contagious. For those with challenges in communication, isolation is an added stressor.

Give psychological support and reassurance to support recovery. Tell the patient they will be warded as soon as it is safe to do so. Monitor your patient for signs of distress and anxiety. If patients become bored and lonely, where possible use technology, such as smart phones and tablets, to maintain communication with relatives and friends, and for patient entertainment.

Activity 5.3 Work-based learning (page 102)

You should ask Mr Woodman when the meal was purchased and how it has been stored. If the meal was purchased the previous evening, even if kept in a domestic fridge, it is unlikely to be safe to eat because rice contains the bacterium Bacillus cereus which can produce gastrointestinal toxins. If it had been purchased on the way to visit the home, within 90 minutes of being cooked, it should be put into a cold store at -5 degrees until it is time to reheat it. The food should be reheated at a temperature above 73 degrees in order to destroy any bacteria. You should use a food temperature probe to ensure it has been heated to the correct temperature. You should record what the food is, where it was purchased and who brought the food into the home, in the event of any untoward occurrence.

Further reading

NHS Standard infection control precautions: essential knowledge and a good place to check your knowledge is up to date. Found at www.england.nhs.uk/patient-safety/standard-infection-control-precautions-national-hand-hygiene-and-personal-protective-equipment-policy/

NICE infection control and prevention quality standards: it covers adults, young people and children and it includes preventing healthcare-associated infections that develop because of treatment, or from being in a healthcare setting. This is found at www.nice.org.uk/guidance/qs61

Rowe et al. (2019) *The Handbook for Nursing Associates and Assistant Practitioners*. London: Sage, Chapter 8.

Useful websites

HSE guidance on fit checking your mask: www.hse.gov.uk/coronavirus/ppe-face-masks/face-mask-ppe-rpe.htm

Sepsis document from the Sepsis Trust: sepsistrust.org/wp-content/uploads/2020/01/5th-Edition-manual-080120.pdf

Best practice guide to food hygiene in care settings. Found at gov.wales/sites/default/files/publications/2019-12/food-and-nutrition-care-homes-older-people-food-hygiene-and-safety.pdf

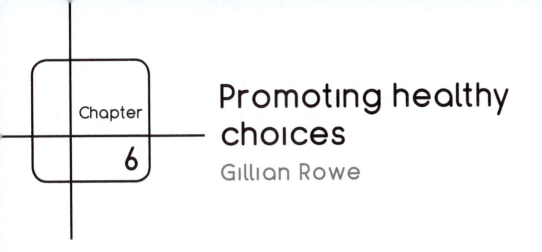

Promoting healthy choices

Gillian Rowe

NMC STANDARDS OF PROFICIENCY FOR NURSING ASSOCIATES

This chapter will address the following platforms and proficiencies:

Platform 2 Promoting health and preventing ill health

2.2   Promote preventive health behaviours and provide information to support people to make informed choices to improve their mental, physical, behavioural health and wellbeing.

Chapter aims

After reading this chapter you will be able to:

1.   use behavioural change models in your practice to promote health choices;
2.   begin conducting motivational interviews;
3.   apply 'making every contact count' to your daily interactions with patients and service users;
4.   determine the factors leading to the need for behaviour change.

Introduction

In 1934, the science fiction writer H.G. Wells, along with his doctor, founded the Diabetics Association. Both had been diagnosed with maturity onset Type 2 diabetes. Frederick Banting and Charles Best had recently created purified insulin (1923) which reduced the death rate; prior to insulin, diabetes killed within a year. Now, the rate at which people develop diabetes is doubling every 20 years and currently 1:15 adults in the UK have diabetes (diabetes.org, 2021). How did we get here? This chapter will explain this.

The NHS long-term plan states 'the NHS will increase its contribution to tackling some of the most significant causes of ill health, including new action to help people stop smoking, overcome drinking problems and avoid Type 2 diabetes, with a particular focus on the communities and groups of people most affected by these problems' (NHS, 2019a). The preferred mechanism for this is an evidence-based approach to improving people's health and wellbeing by helping them change their behaviour (NICE, 2020b). This is, of course, easier said than done. How do we persuade people to abandon unhealthy coping mechanisms and adopt a healthy lifestyle?

This chapter will discuss theoretical models and give you guidance in their application. It will then go on to consider what making every contact count (MECC) is and, equally importantly, what MECC isn't, as defined by HEE. We will then think about motivational interviewing and how to confidently start potentially difficult conversations with people. We will then examine some of the factors that behaviour change addresses by considering the causes and health outcomes of poor lifestyle choices.

One of the first questions to investigate is why people continue to engage in unhealthy behaviours, despite widespread knowledge of the damage that obesity, smoking and excessive alcohol intake can do. For many, these habits are socialised in at a young age and ecological acceptance reinforces them as normalised behaviour. Albert Bandura et al. (1961) developed social learning theory, and this explained that children learn what they live. Older children are also influenced by their peer groups. If an admired peer engages in risky behaviours, other children in the group will also be attracted to those behaviours and copy them.

Once behaviours become established, they are internalised and become part of the individual's identity. By asking someone to change their behaviour, you are also asking them to change their identity, and this can have profound change in their life and relationships. This is especially true where couples both engage in an unhealthy lifestyle and only one wishes to make changes.

Quite often, your patient will have more than one problematic behaviour which needs addressing, such as being an overweight smoker who drinks heavily (Kalkhoran et al., 2018). It takes a very special type of individual to give up more than one behaviour and so your knowledge of your patient will guide you to as to which behaviour needs addressing first. For instance, is their weight the main issue, are they morbidly obese and at risk of Type 2 diabetes (or have developed Type 2 diabetes), or have they developed chronic obstructive pulmonary disease (COPD), or perhaps they have an alcohol-related liver disease (ARLD)? This will indicate the intervention most needed and so you can begin a targeted conversation to promote behaviour change. Activity 6.1 now asks you to explore this problem a little further.

Activity 6.1   Critical thinking and reflection

Effective health promotion is seated within ideas of personalised care and states that generic advice does not work. The patient's own health beliefs will influence their behaviour, but their confidence and **self-belief** in their ability to make and sustain healthy behaviours can impact on whether they are likely to make health promoting adaptions.

How would you go about supporting a patient's confidence? And where would you go to get the information you need?

Suggested answers are at the end of the chapter.

When supporting patients, you need to have a good understanding of local provision. The answer given at the end of the chapter can support you in your knowledge seeking.

Making every contact count (MECC)

Health Education England (HEE) offer training to provide leadership in MECC. This covers instilling confidence in your ability to have brief conversations with patients about health promoting messages and offers prompts to encourage people to make behavioural changes. A link to this training is in the helpful websites section at the end of this chapter.

HEE state that MECC is not about adding another job to already busy working days, but about conversations which take place when you are working with your patients. HEE recognise that staff cannot become specialists or experts in certain lifestyle areas, and nor are they counsellors, but suggest signposting advice and guidance to patients to seek specialist support. They also state that this isn't about staff telling somebody what to do and how to live their life, but offering options to make changes to improve life chances (HEE, 2017). In Activity 6.2, we explore how a student, Sarah, follows HEE advice and consider what she could she have done differently.

Activity 6.2   Communication

MECC:	Student voice: Sarah
	I am currently working at an outreach with women who have suffered domestic abuse. One lady is a heavy smoker with a hacking cough.
Me:	My goodness Mrs B, what are we going to do about your cough?
Mrs B:	What, like giving up smoking?
Me:	Would you like to?
Mrs B:	I'm too stressed to give up.
Me:	It would help to get rid of that cough that keeps you awake. Lack of sleep is bad for stress too.
Mrs B:	I don't think I can.
Me:	Why don't you have a chat with the fag nurse? She can support you and give you some patches.
Mrs B:	I'll think about it.
Me:	Ok, have a think, but if you gave up, you could save enough money to go on that holiday you have been talking about, to reward yourself.
Mrs B:	Yeah, yeah, I could.
Me:	I'll get you some leaflets to read, and you can think about it.

What do you think Sarah did well and what might Sarah have done better?

Compare your answer with the one given at the end of the chapter.

Here, Sarah offered a short intervention of friendly advice and made connections to Mrs B's desire to go on holiday as a goal for positive impetus to change. This follows the NICE explanation of brief interventions as 'ask, advise, assist'.

Understanding the theory

Models of behaviour change

In Chapter 1, we looked at the factors that influence health behaviour and behaviour change. Models of behaviour change recommended by NICE include 'Capability, opportunity and motivation'. This framework states three principles:

1. The individual must be physically and cognitively able to make the change. This means that they have full mental capacity as defined by the Mental Capacity Act (2005) – explored further in Chapter 7 – and are physically able to carry out any recommended activities.
2. The individual must also have physical and social opportunity (so for instance has access to shops which offer healthy or specialised foods).
3. The individual must be motivated to adopt the new behaviour.

This is known as the COM-B model (Michie et al., 2011).

All health promotion interventions should be evidence-based. All the relevant guidelines are contained on the website for the National Institute for Health and Clinical Excellence (NICE). These guidelines offer current best practice in both general and specific situations. The guidance recommends that advice is tailored and sensitive to individual's 'preferences, needs and circumstances' (NICE, 2018).

There are many barriers to an individual adopting health promoting activities, no matter how motivated an individual is. Therefore, it is essential to have a good understanding of your patient's cognitive and physical abilities by discussing with them what changes can be implemented within their limitations. When planning interventions, consider your patient's financial reach. Try not to suggest diets, activities or treatments that are unaffordable.

You should also try to understand your patient's accessibility to affordable good quality food. Many people live in rural areas with only a local corner shop which may carry limited stock. Even in towns and cities, transport may be an issue, not all buses are accessible for wheelchair users. Neither are all railway or London underground stations accessible for those with mobility issues.

Older people or those with cognitive declines might struggle with ordering the weekly shop online. Research by Davidson (2018) has shown that the more elderly your patient is, the less likely they are to be IT literate, and this can be a barrier to accessing interventions.

Motivational interviewing

Helping people change longstanding behaviours that pose health risks is a huge challenge that nursing associates face. Advising people to adopt healthier lifestyles by reducing weight/alcohol/ drugs or by taking prescribed medication can be bewildering when people refuse such advice. It might seem self-evident to you, but many people do not understand the importance or might develop resistance as they feel they are being coerced or made to feel guilty.

Motivational interviewing considers what might inspire change. Prochaska and DiClemente (1986) stated that readiness for change is the vital mediator and suggested that it is a dynamic process. Individuals suffer from ambivalence, swinging from wanting and not wanting to change. Prochaska and DiClemente suggest that people pass through conceptual processes to achieve change (not ready, ready, willing and able). Motivational interviewing is neither authoritarian nor paternalistic: change cannot be achieved by merely telling someone to change.

NICE recommends an individual behaviour change model (NICE, 2018) and states they should be planned using a person-centred approach which takes into account the Equality Act (2010). The key theorists underpinning health promoting practice are Bandura, Antonovsky, Bourdieu and Giddens. These theorists examine self-belief, the **salutinogenic** model, **habitus** and **social reflexivity**. Combining your theoretical knowledge and practical skills brings about praxis, which is the art of caring.

Motivational interviewing is a collaborative process that ensures that the individual's autonomy is respected. Your role is one of facilitating an unmotivated individual to become motivated by discussing the pros and cons of change, by connecting the behaviour to people and things the individual cares about. In Activity 6.1, Sarah knew Mrs B wanted a sunshine holiday abroad and she motivated her thinking by suggesting the money Mrs B spent on cigarettes could be better used for the longed-for break.

Beginning a conversation

As we saw in Chapter 2, when beginning a conversation about change, it is important to think about your body language and paralinguistics: these are pitch, tone and gestures. Ask open ended questions, ask what the individual thinks, and let them take the lead in the conversation. Affirm their statements to give them validation. This will help to build rapport with your patient. Reflect back to the patient to confirm your understanding of what is being said and offer the individual the opportunity to reflect on their thinking. Remember that these are opportunistic conversations. If your patient is worried or particularly unwell, then they should take place another day. Also, you need to make time for conversations to take place. In Activity 6.3, Debbie uses verbal short cuts to move the conversation along.

Case study 6.1

Debbie: I work with the district nursing team, visiting patients in their own home. Sometimes I don't have a lot of time, so I have to use verbal shortcuts.

I will use a verbal Likert Scale when asking patents what changes they would like to make such as 'on a scale of 1 to 10, how important is it for you to make this change, 1 being not important, 10 being very important'.

Then I ask, 'where do we go from here?', so that the patient offers their own solutions to their problems, and I will do my best to support their choices by signposting them to the most appropriate expert or specialist.

Remember: you cannot fix the individual; you can only offer empathy and support their empowerment. The individual must develop commitment to themselves.

Is this something you could adopt in your day-to-day conversations? Would this practice work for you? Reflect on conversations you have had that were time limited.

As this answer is based on your own observation, there is no outline answer at the end of the chapter.

Failure

Many people will have attempted to make a change by themselves but have failed. This will impact their self-efficacy beliefs. Maslow (1943) incorporated self-esteem into his hierarchy of needs. He suggested that there are two forms of self-esteem: self-respect and respect from others. The most important being self-respect, as it is self-protective because it protects the individual against loss of respect from others. Carl Rogers (1961) considered low self-esteem has a relationship with self-worthlessness and feeling incapable of being loved. This can result in the individual not being future orientated, feeling that they have no prospects. This then can then lead to risk taking behaviours and poor lifestyle choices. If you express the belief that a patient is capable of making a change, it will bolster their confidence in trying again.

It is important to remind the individual that falling is not failure but giving up trying is: everyone falls off the wagon and it is important to keep trying.

Obesity

Obesity basically means an individual has a body mass index (BMI) of over 30. Weight management is complex as the causes of obesity are equally complex. There is no single simple answer to weight loss. What is clear is the damage that obesity does to the body, overweight people are prone to metabolic syndrome (obesity, diabetes, hypertension) heart disease, respiratory problems, including sleep disturbance, urinary incontinence, degenerative arthritis (caused by excess weight on the load bearing joints), and cancer. Each of these disorders brings a cascade of associated disorders leading to increased morbidity and avoidable early mortality.

Childhood obesity

Prior to 1970, very few children were obese; 40 years later, many children are. So, what happened in those 40 years? Society has changed enormously; mothers routinely return to the workplace both as a choice and due to economic necessity. The cost of living has increased exponentially. Average wages in 1970 were £130 per month, and an average mortgage was £4,300. This was affordable on a single wage. The average weekly shop was £7.00 per week with a loaf of bread being 9p and a trip to the cinema was 45p. The range of goods available in 1970 was far more restricted than now, there were very few supermarkets (as we understand them now) and purchases were made at the butcher, baker and greengrocer. Britain's love affair with burgers, Indian, Chinese and Italian food was for the future. Fast food came from the fish and chip shop and was a rare treat.

Sweets were an even more occasional treat, usually, or just on a Saturday when pocket money was given in exchange for chores done. Nowadays, to help children's financial literacy, there is an app for that.

Here in 2021, people are time poor. Takeaways and 'ping' micro-meals are often cheaper than the goods needed to create dishes from scratch. Both parents need to work to pay a mortgage or rent, quite often working long hours for minimum wage, and children are bribed with a TV movie, chocolate mini rolls and fizzy drinks to give overwhelmed parents ten minutes peace.

The 1970s child had a bike and played out until dusk. Children now need to be chaperoned everywhere due to perceived (and actual) threats to their safety. Children can no longer play 'in the street' with a long skipping rope or a football as traffic forbids safe play. Public parks and small green areas can often have signs up stating 'No ball games' or 'No skateboarding'. This forces children into passive leisure activities and an energy dense diet.

All these things collaboratively make up what health professionals call 'the **obesogenic environment**'.

In 2019, Professor Dame Sally Davies (ex-CMO) issued a report called 'Time to Solve Childhood Obesity'. She considered the government goal of halving childhood obesity by 2030, suggesting that without a concerted effort, this target would not be met. Her research indicates that in any class of 30 pupils, six children will be obese and a further four will be overweight (Davies, 2019). The approach she recommends considers not just the social determinants of health, as discussed in Chapters 1 and 3, but what she calls the 'commercial determinants of health', recommending that the food industry also contributes to challenging childhood obesity.

Schools play a role in promoting children's health, Ofsted (2018) recently concluded research which examined school's activities in promoting healthy eating and physical activity. School lunches have proved contentious, with people such as Jamie Oliver making public statements (and television programmes) on the standard of food within schools. Ofsted found that up to a quarter of children entering primary education were overweight and that schools, despite their best intentions, were failing to have a measurable impact on reducing childhood obesity. They determined that there were too many factors beyond the school gate which had a greater impact on children's weight.

Parents and caregivers have primary responsibility for monitoring their children's weight, and it is clear that wealth and social class have a role in explaining why children from wealthy families have fewer issues with weight. In the past, it was the rich kids who were fat, which was a sign of parental wealth. The children of the poor were skinny and malnourished. Now, the children of wealthy families are slender. This is a global phenomenon, research by Templin et al. (2019) evidences the incidence of growing obesity in the poorest populations. Their research shows that as poorer nations grow in wealth, the poor are becoming obese. The research documents the change but unhelpfully, does not give any explanation. The availability, quality and affordability of food indicates that reducing childhood obesity requires the combined efforts of government, the food industry, retailers and food educators to have an impact that has lasting effects.

Adult obesity

Modern malnutrition describes the type of malnutrition caused by diets high in sugar, fats and salt. This results in children and adults who are overweight and undernourished in terms of the vitamins and minerals essential for health. Foods which are high in sugar, fats and salt are more likely to be advertised on television and media and promoted within supermarkets at reduced prices. The rise in obesogenic environments includes the prevalence of fast-food takeaways in deprived areas. The combination of low pay, insecure work, high living costs and insufficient state benefits is locking people into poverty. While much is made of the personal responsibility narrative, structural inequality creates a stressful environment that limits food choices.

A lack of health literacy and conflicting advice also hinders the ability of adults to choose wisely. For example, a vegetarian diet is not a reducing diet and needs careful understanding to ensure that vegetarians eat a wide range of foods which offer protein replacement. Vegans need to ensure that they are consuming enough iron, zinc, vitamin D, calcium and omega-3 fatty acid. They are also at risk of developing a vitamin- B12 deficiency which can potentially cause irreversible neurological effects. Older adults suffer declines in taste and smell (Rowe, 2020) and can eat food that is 'off' or add too much salt and sugar to their diet. Also, older adults may have mobility or cognitive issues that can impact their ability to prepare and cook a healthy nutritious meal.

The physiological impact of obesity

We have considered why obesity has increased over the last 50 years and the increase in the obesogenic environment. As stated at the beginning of this section, excess weight stresses the musculo-skeletal system leading to joint degeneration. Also, the proliferating fat cells invade the organs of the immune system, increasing autoimmune disorders such as arthritis. Reduced mobility can exacerbate weight increase leading to the individual becoming immobile and dependent on walking sticks or a wheelchair.

Being overweight and immobile are also causative factors in developing Type 2 diabetes. Type 2 diabetes develops when the body becomes resistant to insulin or when the pancreas is unable to produce enough insulin. Insulin is a hormone that helps to move glucose from the blood stream into cells. If there is an insufficient amount, the glucose remains in the blood stream and makes the blood sticky. This affects the cardiovascular system, so the individual is at higher risk of cardiovascular disease, strokes, heart attacks and diabetic neuropathy.

A strong indication of likelihood of developing diabetes is an individual's Body Mass Index. A BMI of over 35 puts the individual in the obese scale.

Obesity and Covid-19

An international team conducted a meta-analysis of over 300,000 people who were hospitalised due to Covid-19 (SARS-CoV-2) (Rychter et al., 2020). They found that people with obesity (BMI of 35+) were 113 per cent more likely than people of healthy weight to be admitted, 74 per cent more likely to be admitted to an ICU, and 48 per cent more likely to die. These frightening statistics were explained by the physiological effects of obesity.

- Abdominal fat displaces lung capacity and restricts airflow.
- Obese people have a higher tendency for blood clots (Covid-19 injures endothelial cells whose response is to clot blood).
- Obese people have a weakened immune system as fat cells inhabit body organs such as the spleen, bone marrow and thymus, replacing immune tissue with adipose cells.

Also, the very obese suffer from chronic, low-grade inflammation, as fat cells secrete cytokines which may complicate the 'cytokine storm' known in severe Covid-19.

Weight reduction programmes

The UK diet industry is worth approximately £2 billion pounds, with £1.8 billion pounds of specific diet foods sold. There are many commercial products available (Weight Watchers, Slimming World). However, healthy eating advice is offered via the Live Life Well portal (PHE, 2020) and through the 'Change4Life' campaign (NHS, 2020), these websites promote healthy eating behavioural change and are free to access.

The success or otherwise of any reducing diet depends on the determination and commitment of the individual. Research by Madden (2018) for the British Heart Foundation discovered that the average number of days anyone stuck to a diet was 19, whereas it typically takes 66 days to form a new habit. Most overweight people know they should lose a few pounds, but offering weight management advice needs to be handled with tact and diplomacy as it is easy to give offence. Look at Activity 6.4 and consider how you would have handled the interaction Brianna has with her patient.

Activity 6.3   Reflection

Making every contact count: Student Nursing Associate Brianna

I was supporting Mrs Brown to take her diabetes medication when I mentioned that I was putting on weight and needed to go on a diet. Mrs Brown said she needed to too. I took this as a good moment to discuss the benefits of weight loss on Type 2 diabetes.

If you were Brianna, what advice would you give to Mrs Brown? Reflect and jot down your thoughts.

Compare your thoughts with the suggested answers at the end of the chapter.

Brianna could suggest that Mrs Brown join a slimming club if her doctor were agreeable. Mrs Brown would need to be careful which diet she embarked upon. Many commercial diets have 'fast starts' but these are not intended to last longer than four weeks. Intermittent fasting and low-carbohydrate diets are popular with some limited supporting evidence-based research. This approach to weight loss is effective but should not be undertaken by people with diabetes or by pregnant or breast-feeding mothers without medical supervision.

What is a healthy diet?

The standard advice is to eat a diet rich in vegetables, fruits, legumes, lean protein, seeds and nuts, and healthy snacks. Also, to avoid sugar-rich fizzy drinks, although natural fruit juices are high in sugar, they can be diluted, and squashes are now sugar free. Processed foods are high in unhealthy fats, salt and sugar and should be avoided.

The NHS offers the 'Eatwell plate' as a guide to the proportions of various foods. Eating smaller portions helps. However, plate sizes have undergone a huge transformation in the last

40 years. A dinner plate in your grandparents' time was not a lot bigger than a side plate is now. A standard dinner plate was 9 inches with a 1.5 inch rim. Plates are now 12 inches or bigger and the same can be found with pudding bowls. Much larger tableware can lead to much larger portions and add 7 lbs a year to an individual's weight. An effective suggestion for weight loss could be changing tableware.

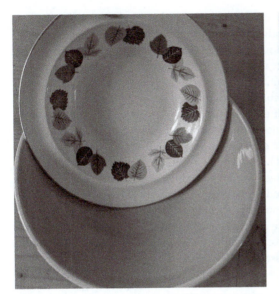 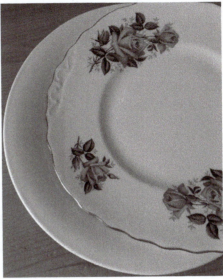

Figure 6.1 Photographs of comparative plates and bowls

Smoking cessation

In the 1950s, the relationship between tobacco smoke and lung cancer was confirmed. It took until the mid-1960s before tobacco advertising was banned and anti-smoking adverts appeared in media and on television. Smoking is discouraged by the use of progressive taxation and restriction on the places where people can smoke (public transport, pubs and restaurants), and smoking in cars where children are present is also banned. Smoking is now stigmatised throughout the western world. Graham (2012) said, 'Being a smoker has become a stigmatized identity linked inextricably to other stigmatized identities (for example, to "welfare mother" in the United States and "chav" in the United Kingdom)'.

Smoking prevalence has declined year on year since 2011 (ONS, 2020a) with an average fall of 0.6 per cent annually. In 2018, 14.7 per cent of the population smoked. In 2019, it was 14.1 per cent. There are slight differences between the countries that make up the United Kingdom. In Wales and Scotland, 15.5 per cent of the population smoke, in Northern Ireland it is 15.6 per cent and in England 13.9 per cent of the population are smokers (ONS, 2020a).

Smoking has a socio-economic distribution, those in the lowest socio-economic groups are more likely to smoke than those in the professions. Unemployed people are also more likely to smoke, as are those who are divorced, widowed or single. Ethnic minorities such as Black, Chinese and Muslim men are more likely to smoke, but minority women are much less likely to smoke suggesting that there is a cultural element to smoking acceptability (ONS, 2020a).

Support for smoking cessation

Many smokers state that they wish to stop smoking, however, overcoming tobacco addiction requires determination and usually takes many attempts. The NHS states that 'Smoking is a relapsing addiction, and many people have 6–7 attempts before quitting long term' (NHS, 2020). Backsliding is often caused by stressful life events as new non-smokers have yet to develop healthier coping mechanisms.

A Cochrane review of smoking cessation methods (Lindson et al., 2019) revealed that 'cutting down' (preparing to stop) was no more effective than going cold turkey (stopping smoking all at once) and that pharmacological intervention was generally needed for the stop attempt to be effective. There are easy-to-purchase nicotine replacement therapy patches, lozenges, gum and sprays available in supermarkets and pharmacies. Short-term medication such as varenicline (Champix) and Bupropion (Zyban) are available on prescription, however, these have noted off target side effects, and neither are suitable or effective for all.

The NHS stop smoking service offers a wide range of support, based in communities. Usually, a specialist stop-smoking nurse is available in each GP surgery or pharmacy. These services are free with both one to one and group sessions held within the local community.

Individuals attending smoking cessation sessions are given a breath test, which measures the amount of carbon monoxide in their breath and a prescription or vouchers are given for nicotine replacement therapy. People giving up smoking are given counselling regarding weight gain and how to develop healthy coping mechanisms to support them through adverse events. You might consider Activity 6.5, as this could be a collaborative activity with your fellow trainees and would evidence your understanding of smoking cessation.

Activity 6.4 Work-based learning

You could run your own 'Stoptober' campaign either at your university or workplace. PHE Stoptober resources are freely available to download and print off to display and flyers to hand out. You would need to discuss this with your college tutor or your workplace supervisor to ensure you have their permission and cooperation.

Find resources here: campaignresources.phe.gov.uk/resources/campaigns/6-stoptober/resources

This activity does not have a provided answer as it is work-based learning.

Online support

The NHS have several apps in the NHS app store and those who wish to stop smoking should be directed to try them. However, those who have cognitive deficits or physical disabilities may be excluded from smartphone support. Also, as stated earlier in the chapter, older smokers may not be IT literate, own a smart phone or have internet provision, and this is a major barrier to access.

The National Centre for Smoking Cessation and Training (NCSCT) has developed a short training module on how to deliver 'Very Brief Advice on Smoking'. This training module is built around evidence-based behaviour change techniques that provide an understanding of the factors involved in smoking and smoking cessation. The training programme has been shown to increase practitioners' knowledge, develop their skills and lead to improved practice. You could engage in this module if you are attempting Activity 6.5.

Promoting healthy ageing: slips, trips and falls

Managing elderly care health promotion involves falls prevention. Falls are a common issue for those over 65 years of age, with half of those aged over 80 falling several times a year (Fenton, 2017). The impact of broken bones (especially neck of the femur) on quality of life is significant. Older people do not always notice that their physical health is deteriorating and may not understand that impaired vision and deafness have an impact on balance. A previous fall is an indicator of likely future falls. This is probably because environmental issues have not been addressed or because fear of falling has reduced the individual's physical activity, leaving them physically weaker.

Falls factors

The main risk factors for the likelihood of someone having a fall are strength, gait or balance. These can be exacerbated by an individual having osteoporosis or vitamin D deficiency, and impaired vision.

Various types of medication such as sedatives (sleeping pills) and anti-depressants have been indicated in morning falls.

Use of diuretics and dehydration can lead to dizziness. Fear of incontinence results in rushing to the toilet which can cause trips and falls. Low blood pressure (hypotension) and low blood sugar (hypoglycaemia) can cause dizziness.

People suffering some chronic conditions such as stroke, Parkinson's and Alzheimer's are more likely to suffer falls as cognitive declines reduce hazard perception.

Footwear has also been indicated, with loose (floppy) slippers a prime candidate for trips and slips.

Post-menopausal women are at greater risk of fragility fractures of the wrist, hips and spine due to osteoporosis, as the protection given by oestrogen slowly ebbs. They may also be a familial component as osteoporosis tends to run in families (The Royal Osteoporosis Society, 2020).

Drugs such as steroids and anti-epilepsy medication also have an influence on bone density. Other contributing factors include very low body weight, smoking, high alcohol intake, diabetes and a diet lacking in calcium and vitamin D.

Difficulty getting into and out of the bath or shower can lead to falls and sometimes people can remain in the bath or on the floor of the bathroom for some significant time before help comes, and as a consequence, suffer from hypothermia. Activity 6.6 asks you to think about assessing a candidate for slips, trips and falls.

Activity 6.5   Critical thinking

While working on a ward with an occupational therapist, Ellis is approached by 76-year-old Mr Chen. Mr Chen tells Ellis that he is a bit wobbly on his feet.

How would Ellis evaluate Mr Chen as a likely trip candidate? What advice would you give to Ellis?

Later, Ellis is engaged in a home assessment for Mr Chen. If you were to write a checklist for him, what would you include? Think about likely hazards around the home.

Suggested answers are at the end of the chapter.

Psychological impact

Mr Chen's age is a factor in his likelihood of falling, as is his statement to Ellis that he is a bit 'wobbly', he is at risk of developing a fear of falling. People who have had a fall tend to develop a fear of falling and this impacts on their psychological wellbeing. This can impact their self-belief and self-efficacy and compromise their quality of life and their ability to have an independent life. Developing dependence on others to do the tasks they have always performed can lead to a sense of guilt, of being a burden, leading to embarrassment and anxiety. Loss of confidence can lead to timidity and refusing to participate in social activities. Fear of falling can be more debilitating in the long run, than the original fall.

Promoting fitness

NHS advice for healthy ageing is to engage is strength building activities such as ball games, racquet games, circuit training, resistance training and Nordic walking. Knowledge of local community provision will help you in the advice you give, as there may well be keep fit clubs for the elderly, U3A (University of the Third Age) walking groups, swimming or water-based fitness activities available.

The cost of slips, trips and falls to the NHS is annually approximately £3 billion, with approximately 5 per cent of falls requiring surgical intervention. Public Health England reported that from 2017 to 2018 there were around 220,160 emergency hospital admissions related to falls among patients aged 65 and over, with around 146,665 (66.6 per cent) of these patients aged 80 and over. See Table 6.1 from PHE (2019) which indicates the number of falls per 100,000 per head of population within the regions.

Table 6.1   Number of falls

Recent trends:	Could not be calculated	No significant change	⬆ Increasing and getting worse	⬆ Increasing and getting better	⬇ Decreasing and getting worse	⬇ Decreasing and getting better
Indicator			Period	England count	England value	Recent trend
Emergency hospital admissions due to falls in people aged 65 and over			2019/20	234,793	2,222 per 100,000	⬆
Emergency hospital admissions due to falls in people aged 65–79			2019/20	77,427	1,042 per 100,000	⬆
Emergency hospital admissions due to falls in people aged 80+			2019/20	157,366	5,644 per 100,000	⬆

Individually, 40 per cent of those suffering a fractured hip will die within six months of surgery and a further 15 per cent will die within a year. Therefore, falls prevention will save lives and money.

Alcoholism and problem drinking

Alcoholism, or AUD (Alcohol Use Disorder), includes both physical and psychological addiction to alcohol. People who develop alcoholism often are not aware that their drinking has become problematic. It is only when their drinking affects their work, home, relationships and finances that they recognise that their drinking is an issue. If drinking takes a precedence over all the other activities of daily living and the individual experiences withdrawal symptoms such as nausea, sweating or shaking when they are not drinking, then they clearly have a dependence.

Chronic alcoholism can cause cardiovascular diseases, pancreatitis, liver disease including cirrhosis, gastric ulcers, osteoporosis, foetal alcohol syndrome, peripheral neuropathy and complicate diabetes. It can also cause blackouts, psychosis and paranoia.

Problem drinking

Binge drinking (heavy episodic drinking) is a patten of excessive alcohol intake (eight or more drinks) in a short time period. People drinking in this manner are drinking to get drunk. They are at risk of alcohol poisoning, falls and accidents. Alcohol depresses the nerves that control involuntary actions such as the gag reflex which prevent choking, so those who are very drunk can die by asphyxiation due to vomit inhalation. Also, an alcohol overdose can lead to irreversible brain damage.

The current fad for downing 'shots' over a short period of time can lead to violence (physical and sexual assault), unwanted pregnancy, STIs and images appearing on social media that can damage career prospects.

Treatment

Alcohol withdrawal needs professional support, medical detoxification is usually undertaken in specialist units. Home treatment is possible with medication such as naltrexone, disulfiram, nalmefene or acamprosate, which are used to prevent relapse. Chlordiazepoxide is a tranquilliser which is effective for withdrawal side effects. Local support is given by regular visits from a healthcare professional and professional extended counselling. For alcoholics, lifelong abstinence is often the goal as a single drink can lead to resurgence of the addiction.

For those wishing to cut down (moderation rather than abstinence), brief intervention is offered (lasting about ten minutes) and examines drinking habits and what support networks are available locally. Patients will usually be offered CBT to help with any psychological issues which might be driving the excess drinking.

Alcoholism doesn't just affect the drinker: it affects families too. Therefore, support for the family is available, Al-Anon is a support agency that offers advice for relatives and friends. The web address is at the end of the chapter if you wanted to research further.

Illegal street drugs

Illegal drugs that are available to purchase have a variability in purity, they can be mixed with diluents which are intended to bulk out the content or by adulterants which are intended to enhance the effects. By virtue of being illegal, the purchaser has no real idea of what they are buying or the effect until they take the drug.

County lines

The recent phenomena of 'county lines' is the means whereby organised drug criminals pressurise vulnerable people such as drug addicts, or people who are vulnerable due to mental or physical health impairments, single mothers, sex workers and children to transport, store and sell drugs in smaller county towns. Vulnerable people are coerced into using their homes to store and deal drugs (cuckooing).

Vulnerable children are given drugs to sell within senior schools and youth facilities or they may be used as 'mules' to carry drugs across counties (hence the name). Once entrapped, children are subject to abuse, sexual violence and exploitation. Research by the Children's Society (Counting Lives, 2019) evidenced that children as young as seven, but usually teenagers, are recruited by grooming to supply illegal drugs.

Problem drug users

Problem drug users are also likely to have other health problems, especially people who inject drugs (PWID). The likelihood of developing blood borne diseases due to needle sharing includes hepatitis B and C, HIV/AIDS and bacterial endocarditis. PHE (2020) states that 48 per cent of addicts are unaware of having hepatitis. They are also more likely to suffer malnutrition, lung disorders and dental problems.

Needle and syringe programmes (NSPs) are available from pharmacies and drug outreach workers. They often supply sterile water also. Some pharmacies also supply oral Methadone (and other recovery targeted drugs). Local provision depends on population density. Rural locations tend to have fewer local facilities.

If someone does disclose to you that they are drug user, you should signpost them to a drugs professional who can tailor advice to the person's preferences, needs and level of understanding about their health.

Promote your own health: taking care of yourself

Resilience is something that features in nursing associates' contracts. You are required to engage in self-care activities and learn how to protect your own mental health.

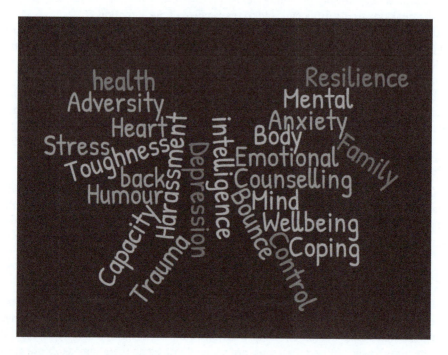

Figure 6.2   Resilience word cloud

Resilience describes the ability to bounce back from situations which can lead to poor mental health. Being under continuous stress can lead to distress. If you are continually exposed to stressful situations this can lead to anxiety and depression. Despite resilience being a current cultural buzzword, it can offer solutions to stress. The working environment for nursing associates makes a huge demand on physical and mental resources and has led to many members of staff leaving nursing for less challenging work. Staff and resource shortfalls are a major factor in workplace stress.

There are activities you can engage in that are mentally protective.

1. The first, best and hardest is getting a good night's sleep, stress hormones such as cortisol and epinephrine (adrenaline) prevent sleep, the fight or flight hormones prepare your body for action and are not conducive to rest. If you have had a stressful day, the best way to rid your body of these is to walk or run them off. If this is not possible, have a relaxing bath or long shower. The benefits of relaxation are that it gives you the opportunity to reflect on your day and determine why it was so stressful and what opportunities there are for reducing the stress. The better quality of sleep you get, the more you are able to deal with challenges at work.

2. Employers can be consulted as to how pattens of work can be better organised. Long shifts and sequence of shifts can be modified to reduce continuous workloads, for instance, changing to shift pattens to those that are health protective.

3. Take your breaks. You cannot help people if you are hungry, thirsty or want to use the toilet. Fifteen minutes away from work gives you the chance to attend to your needs.

4. Practice negative thought restructuring: get your internal voice under control and maintain a perspective on the day's events. Build your self-esteem by thinking more about your strengths than your weaknesses.

5. Build your self-confidence through knowledge acquisition and praxis. Use reflection to identify any gaps and talk to your supervisor about how to address them. Do not engage in activities that you are not confident about; it is better to refuse than make an error.

6. Be flexible. Change happens; embrace the changes and work with them. If you can develop a 'can do' attitude and adopt a proactive problem-solving attitude you will feel more in control.

7. Support your team. Develop a network of supportive colleagues for a collaborative approach to problem solving. They can also act as a sounding board for your ideas and offer a shoulder to cry on if you are feeling overwhelmed.

8. Learn from your mistakes. Every mistake you make is an opportunity to understand the notion of post traumatic growth. Use reflection to understand how mistakes are made and how you can improve, but do not blow events out of proportion.

9. When you are away from work, do not dwell on work-related stuff. Chat to friends and family, take time out and enjoy your day off.

Chapter summary

This chapter has discussed the ways you can use models of behaviour change to engage in MECC. It has provided you with learning opportunities and websites for you to visit to enhance your knowledge of obesity and diet, healthy ageing, smoking cessation, alcoholism, illegal drugs and taking care of yourself.

Activities: brief outline answers

Activity 6.1 Critical thinking and reflection (page 106)

Burd and Halsworth (2016) state that there are three elements to influencing behaviour change: the capability of the patent, their motivation and the opportunity to make changes. By understanding a patient's readiness to change, supportive empowering and sensitive coaching can enhance the patient's self-efficacy. To support your patients, you should have an understanding of provision so you can point to specific organisations both locally and nationally. Most helpful organisations have a website, and some have locality offices.

What is available in your locality? You will need local knowledge of helping organisations:

- where the clinics are held to support smoking cessation;
- local provision to support poor mental health or offer affordable cognitive behavioral therapy (CBT);
- affordable weight loss programmes;
- alcohol withdrawal programmes.

Most county council websites hold this information. Look up yours and make a list of contacts for your future use.

Activity 6.2 Communication (page 107)

Sarah's MECC was friendly and evidenced her understanding of her client. She initially followed HEE advice but then pre-empted the smoking cessation nurse as to possible interventions. This was inappropriate. Interventions are planned between the smoking cessation nurse and the patient.

Activity 6.3 Reflection (page 112)

Brianna could have told Mrs Brown that losing 15 kgs of weight would support diabetes remission, that she would have more energy and her mobility would improve. It would also lower her blood pressure and reduce her cholesterol count; this would also reduce her risk of a heart attack and a stroke (cerebrovascular accident).

Activity 6.5 Critical thinking (page 115)

Ellis could ask Mr Chen if he has fallen at all this year. If so, he has an increased likelihood of falling again. Ellis should be proactive, observing Mr Chen walking and check for pace, gait, sway and balance. He should note any concerns and ensure this is communicated to the team within the patient notes.

To evaluate likely trip candidates 'Timed up and go' is a quick and easy assessment tool. Sit your patient on a standard chair, ask your patient to stand up, walk five paces, turn around, walk back and sit down again. Time them; if they take more than 12 seconds, they are at risk of falls.

MECC: Ellis could offer a copy of the leaflet: *Get Up and Go: A Guide to Staying Steady*. This can be found at www.csp.org.uk/publications/get-go-guide-staying-steady-english-version to download and print off copies.

Trip hazards in the home: How many of these did you include? Mats, frayed carpet, poor lighting, trailing cables, loose staircase treads, items left on the floor, unsteady furniture (casters or wobbly legs), height of the bed (too high or too low), bedside lighting, staircase handrails, grab rails in the bathroom, non-slip bathroom and kitchen flooring, uneven or slippery paving in the garden. Reach and bend could also be an issue when people access high or low cupboards.

Further reading

Health Promotion: Planning and Strategies 4th edition (2019; by Green, Cross, Woodall and Tones. London: SAGE) is a useful textbook for planning intervention strategies. It is useful because it acknowledges the social dimension in health promotion.

Communicating Health: Strategies for Health Promotion (2013; by Corcoran. London: SAGE). Although this is an older book, it offers useful critique of the theoretical models currently used.

Foundations for Health Promotion (2016; by Naidoo and Wills. London: Elsevier) is a good general textbook and excellent as a foundation text to enhance understanding of the basics of health promotion.

Useful websites

Free MECC training can be found here: www.e-lfh.org.uk/programmes/making-every-contact-count/. If you do not have an NHS login, you can still access the training, but you will not get a certificate.

The NHS Eatwell plate: www.nhs.uk/live-well/eat-well/the-eatwell-guide/

Alcoholics anonymous: www.alcoholics-anonymous.org.uk/

County lines: www.nationalcrimeagency.gov.uk/what-we-do/crime-threats/drug-trafficking/county-lines

The RCN has resilience guides you can read at www.rcn.org.uk/library/subject-guides/wellbeing-self-care-and-resilience. You do not need to be a member to access them. The NHS also offers guidance: www.england.nhs.uk/wp-content/uploads/2016/03/releas-capcty-6-topic-sht-6-2.pdf

MECC: very brief advice training session for smoking cessation: www.ncsct.co.uk/publication_very-brief-advice.php

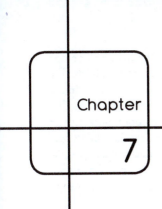

Chapter 7

Promoting good mental health

Gillian Rowe

Chapter aims

This chapter will introduce you to some fundamental theoretical knowledge of mental health. After reading this chapter you will be able to:

1.   examine notions of stigma, prejudice, and stereotyping;
2.   discuss the major theoretical perspectives;
3.   consider the legal and policy frameworks;
4.   examine the classification of mental health;
5.   identify mental health promotion activities.

According to the World Health Organization (WHO, 2018b), good mental health can be understood as 'a state of well-being in which the individual realizes his or her own abilities, can cope with the normal stresses of life, can work productively and fruitfully, and is able to make a contribution to his or her own community' and this conceptual definition will be this chapter's working model.

It is an arresting but true statistic that one in four people will experience poor mental health at some point in their lives. Look around your staff room or your classroom, there will be people there who have or who are experiencing mental ill health. You too, might be one of those people. Health professionals are great at sharing physical ill health stories, but we seldom share poor mental health stories. Why is poor mental health so stigmatised? Why are the words we use to describe poor mental health so derogatory? Let us explore further.

Introduction

The causes of poor mental health are many, varied and can be caused by a combination of circumstances: childhood and adult emotional or physical trauma, bereavement, long term stress, chronic physical ailments, unemployment, or insecure work, insecure low wage and resultant poverty; homelessness, risk of homelessness and living in a home unfit for habitation; social isolation, discrimination and stigma. Some forms of mental ill health may be familial (inherited) and some are culturally mediated (different cultures have a different understanding or explanation for behaviours).

The main problem with mental ill health is that it seldom has any physical manifestation (unless it results from a physiological disorder such as tertiary syphilis or Alzheimer's disease). Therefore, it reveals itself through behaviours (signs), thoughts and feelings (symptoms). The context or circumstance of the behaviour will determine how much (or little) the behaviour is tolerated by society. This is called deviation from socio-cultural norms. Some cultures are more tolerant, others less so.

Historically, poor mental health thought to be caused by supernatural agents such as evil spirits, witches spells or possession by demons. Trepanning was performed by drilling a hole in the skull to let the devils out, an early form of psychosurgery. This theory was displaced by somatogenic theories, the idea that the body's humours (black and yellow bile, blood, and phlegm) were out of balance and was remedied by phlebotomy (bleeding the patient). This too was superseded, replaced by psychogenic theories which focused on trauma and stress.

For the Georgians and early Victorians, poor mental health indicated either bad blood (inherited characteristics) or a lack of self-control. Such patients were incarcerated into asylums. These forbidding structures were places of terror. Patients were treated as animals, chained to the walls or locked in cells. Eventually, late Victorian activists persuaded authorities to be more humane and offer therapeutic interventions. Patients were encouraged to participate in art and nature and were treated with a degree of dignity and courtesy.

Philosophical meditations on the causes of mental ill health led inevitably to the nature-versus-nurture debate. Whether mental disorders have a predominant biological cause or if parenting, trauma or other social and environmental agencies are the cause.

You will notice, as we go through the chapter, that these historical notions reappear, modernised, but still recognisable.

Parity of esteem

The Mental Health Foundation defines parity of esteem as 'valuing mental health equally with physical health', this means equal access to effective treatment and care. Adult mental health has always been considered a 'Cinderella service' less attractive work with limited funding. The government's (Department of Health and Social Care, 2011) policy document 'No Health without

Mental Health' signalled an acknowledgment that mental health provision was fragmented and piecemeal. Parity of esteem was enshrined in the Health and Social Care Act (2012), and the 'NHS Five Years Forward for Mental Health' plan made six recommendations to achieve parity of esteem. The intention is to achieve a more holistic service that considers both physical and mental health in care planning. Mental ill health and physical ill health are treated as separate entities, whereas the reality is that they have a reciprocal relationship: chronic pain affects mental health, and poor mental health can affect somatic disorders.

Martin McShane, writing in 2013, stated:

Let me give you some facts; over 75% of those with heart disease are in treatment, for people with diabetes or hypertension more than 90% are in treatment. Conversely only 25% of people with depression or anxiety receive treatment. If you have mental illness, it can reduce your life expectancy by 10 years because of your poor physical health, individuals with mental health issues have the same life expectancy as the general population did 50 years ago.

Eight years later, very little has changed. Although 'Next Steps on Five Year Forwards for Mental Health' state that the NHS introduced and met national wait times for mental health services (england.nhs, 2016), recent research by the Royal College of Psychiatrists found that two-fifths of patients waiting for mental health treatment were forced to resort to emergency or crisis services and that nearly two-thirds (64 per cent of those surveyed) waited more than four weeks between their initial assessment and second appointment, some waited between six and eleven months (RCPsch, 2020). The King's Fund research indicates that lack of funding provision for clinical commissioning groups (CCG) and workforce shortages have contributed to a lack of service provision.

Stigma, stereotyping and discrimination

Stigma arose from fears of the insane. Lack of knowledge of causation, the fear of contagion and fear of unpredictability in behaviour led to exclusion from society. Melancholia (depression) was viewed as a personal failing and therefore not deserving of sympathy or support. Shrivastava et al. (2012) state that 'Causes and consequences of stigma are often indistinguishable and lead to prejudices that influence attitudes, which in turn increase prejudices perpetually'. Ervine Goffman, a Canadian social psychologist, wrote extensively on notions of a 'spoilt identity'. He described it as the 'situation of the individual who is disqualified from full social acceptance' (Goffman, 1963).

Goffman noted that people with poor mental health had 'stigmatised identities', meaning that the individual is devalued by society and discredited due to their ill health. Goffman explained that sufferers were susceptible to discrimination and that stigmatization is an interactive social process. The sufferer experienced 'felt' stigma, we would now call this 'self' stigma. The desire not to be negatively labelled can prevent people from accessing care and support when they need it. Professor Kay Jamison Redfield, a psychologist who has bipolar disorder, said

It was difficult to make the decision to be public about having a severe psychiatric illness ... but privacy and reticence can kill. The problem with mental illness is that so many who have it – especially those in a position to change public attitudes, such as doctors, lawyers, politicians, and military officers – are reluctant to risk talking about mental illness or seeking help for it. They are understandably frightened about professional and personal reprisals.

(Redfield, Jamison, 2001)

Stereotypes can come from media depictions; media can influence perceptions of mental health and serve as a socialising influence when others are absent. Media, such as television, film and social media, such as YouTube and Instagram, contribute to mental health stigma through exaggerated, inaccurate and comic images. Mind Researchers found that 66 per cent of mental ill health portrayals on UK television focused on violent and unpredictable behaviours. Such negative media representations increase people's mental distress through self-stigma and can lead to social isolation.

Activity 7.1   Critical thinking

Unfortunately, not all conditions are treated equally in the media. Mental health problems such as depression, anxiety and bipolar disorder are starting to be treated with sympathy and understanding on screen. However, when schizophrenia and personality disorders are covered it is usually in connection to violence, even though we know that you're much more likely to be a victim than a perpetrator of violence if you have a mental health problem.

(Jenni Regan Mind Senior Media Advisor)

Think about the television programmes and films you have watched recently; how do they portray mental ill health? how do they compare with attitudes to mental health portrayed in past films such as *One Flew Over the Cuckoo's Nest*? Would you agree or disagree with Jenni Regan, do you think media portrayal is improving?

As this is a personal reflection on the programmes you have watched, there is no given answer.

Intersectionality theory explains why children and adults with multiple layers of social disadvantage can experience discrimination and oppression (see Chapter 8). Factors such as disability, race, sexual orientation, gender and poverty can combine to intensify stigma and the development of a stigmatised identity. The sociocultural perspective considers people's behaviours and mental processes which are shaped in part by their social and cultural contexts (cultural relativism), including race, gender and nationality. Ethnic minorities have traditionally been reluctant to engage with mental health services as they fear cultural stigma. Different cultures describe or explain their feelings in ways which can lead to misunderstanding. Finding a mental health professional who understands those specific experiences, traditions and concerns is difficult. Lack of language fluency can also impact on access to mental health services and affect the individuals' understanding of health terminology.

People who experience poor mental health are often discriminated against or have stereotypical labels applied which allow discrimination to take place. Young people who suffer anorexia nervosa or who self-harm are labelled 'attention seekers' (Farooq, 2019), and their psychological distress is marginalised or dismissed. This reflects the Victorian notion that poor mental health is a lack of self-control and the sufferer is deviant and unworthy. However, this attitude can have consequence, anorexia nervosa has the highest mortality rate of any psychiatric disorder in adolescence (NICE, 2020a).

Major theoretical approaches to mental health

There are seven major theoretical approaches to understanding mental health.

1. analytical/psychodynamic: the main theorists are Freud and Jung;
2. developmental theories: the main theorists are Eriksson and Kohlberg;

3. cognitive theories: the main theorists are Chomsky, Piaget and Tolman;
4. behavioural theories: the main theorists are Pavlov, Skinner and Watson;
5. the humanist approach: the main theorists are Maslow and Rogers;
6. social psychology theories: the main theorists are Bandura, Festinger and Lewin;
7. the trauma model: the main theorists are Ross, Athens and R. D. Laing.

Three of these disparate theories were (to some extent) united by the biopsychosocial model, devised by George Engel in 1977. It is both a philosophy of care and a clinical guide which offers a more holistic approach than the prevailing biomedical model. Engel's approach was designed to include the patient's perspective on their ailment and offered empowerment for the individual. Engel stated that 'The patient–clinician relationship influences medical outcomes, even if only because of its influence on adherence to a chosen treatment' (Engel, 1980).

The biopsychosocial approach has been juxtaposed with the biopsychiatric model which re-emerged in the early 2000s. It is considered as a psychiatric response in support of the biomedical model. This biological model uses molecular biology to examine the brain's structure and function as the focus of poor mental health. Researchers seek biomarkers or genetic abnormalities for specific mental disorders. Researchers have had successes with understanding how Alzheimer's disease progresses, and have found evidence of genetic components for schizophrenia, bipolar disorder and autism. Further research has clarified how medication interacts with neurotransmitters in the treatment of anxiety, depression, schizophrenia and attention deficit disorder. This will hopefully, lead to new biologic medications which targets specific faulty genes or gene combinations.

Anti-psychiatry

The biopsychiatric model also reflects the Victorian notion of 'bad blood' being the cause of poor mental health and has been critiqued in the past by such as Thomas Szasz, R. D. Laing and Michel Foucault. Szasz and Laing were part of the 'anti-psychiatry' movement, led by psychiatrists who felt that treatment was more damaging than the original disorder, and that mental health diagnosis lacked scientific validity. Niall McLaren (2007) considers the biopsychiatric model to be reductionist (reducing people to the sum of their biological components, like the components that make up a machine) and he considers this model does not have a theory of the mind and so rejects personality, environmental experience and the human spirit.

Spiritual model

The artificial division of physical health from mental health adopted in western medicine, courtesy of René Descartes, is not shared by traditional cultures. Physical and mental health has long been deemed as being related to the emotional, social or spiritual health of the person. We would call this a holistic or spiritual model.

Spiritual beliefs are not automatically tied to any particular religious belief or culture. Whilst each religion has its own traditions and rituals, spirituality can be a personal experience for anyone, with or without a religious belief. Prayer and meditation are similar and share characteristics with mindfulness. Being part of a spiritual community can bring peace, hope and a sense of continuity. Spiritual people often feel part of something bigger than themselves and may feel strength in fellowship.

Some religious conventions can help in times of mental confusion, but others can harm. Especially those religions which believe poor mental health is a form of possession by demons, harking back to medieval practices, such as exorcism. These practices may prevent vulnerable unwell people from seeking professional help.

Medication

The pharmacologic revolution of the 1950s developed new drugs to relieve poor mental health. Prior to pharmacology, surgical intervention in the form of the lobotomy (leucotomy in America) was an accepted form of intervention, along with malarial therapy, insulin shock therapy, cardiozol shock therapy and electro-convulsive therapy (ECT). Most of these interventions have been discredited, ECT remains a treatment option for severe depressive illness, catatonia or a prolonged manic episode, although now steadily declining in use.

Psychotropic medication was and is predicated on behavioural pharmacology. The search and research for drugs which altered behaviours did not always follow ethical standards and was at times misguided. Drugs were created to improve the management of disease and used before there was any clear understanding of how the drugs actually worked. These drugs assumed an imbalance of the hormones released by neurotransmitters (such as adrenaline, serotonin, etc.) was the cause of psychosis (rather like the notion of imbalance of the humours). And that by making chemical adjustments, the patient would be returned to normality. Many patients were harmed in the process of discovering how drugs worked.

Ivan Illich coined the phrase 'iatrogenesis' in his work *Medical Nemesis* (1975) to describe medicine induced ailments. He considered many interventions to be ineffective, toxic or unsafe and his work triggered the need for evidence-based practice. The pharmacological industry has been slow to adopt safe, ethical practice although it has made some progress in the intervening years. However, adverse drug reactions and off target side effects still cause between 5 and 8 per cent of all deaths worldwide (Peer and Shabir, 2018).

There are five classifications of psychotropic drugs:

1. antipsychotics: such as Aripiprazole and Olanzapine;
2. antidepressants: such as Sertraline and Citalopram;
3. anxiolytics: such as Clonazepam and Diazepam;
4. hypnotics: such as Flurazepam and Eszopiclone;
5. mood stabilisers: such as Carbamazepine and Lamotrigine.

However, some drugs can be used in more than one classification depending on dose, such as Quetiapine which can be used as an antipsychotic, antidepressant, hypnotic and a mood stabiliser.

All drugs carry side effects from the mild (thirst, itch, nausea, constipation, weight gain) to serious problems such as cardiac disturbances, fatigue and abnormal face and body movements. They also cause (thankfully rare) medical emergencies such as anaphylaxis, neuroleptic malignant syndrome and serotonin syndrome.

Classification of mental ailments

Mental ill health is defined by criteria contained in the American Diagnostic and Statistical Manual of Mental Disorders (DSM). This covers all categories of mental health disorders for both adults and children, and it describes the symptoms necessary for diagnosis. The DSM originated within the American health insurance system and the need for categorisation for the payment of medical bills.

Commenced in 1952, it had 102 diagnoses, the latest edition DSM-IV-TR-5 (2013), contains 365 diagnoses. This was published with considerable controversy as many of the contributing psychiatrists had financial relationships with pharmaceutical companies. Other criticism includes the arbitrary nature of the cut offs between normal and pathological. Also critiqued was a lack of cultural differentiation as cultures differ quite significantly in their conception of normality. What is considered 'normal' in one culture can be considered 'abnormal' or 'pathological' in another one (Francis, 2013). There is a view that this subjectivity is not scientific, particularly as mental health diagnosis carries risk to the individual in terms of over medication and social stigma.

The other disease classification system is the International Classification of Disease (ICD). The latest edition is ICD-11 which officially takes effect in January 2022, and it is hosted by the World Health Organization (WHO). WHO state it is 'the international standard for systematic recording, reporting, analysis, interpretation and comparison of mortality and morbidity data' (WHO, 2018d); however, the DSM only covers mental ill health diagnosis whereas the ICD covers physical and mental disorders and collects and collates international morbidity and mortality statistics.

The legal and policy framework

Mental health legislation has a long history, generally in regard to incarceration. The main pieces of current legislation you need to understand is the Mental Health Act 1983 (and 2007 amendments) and the Mental Capacity Act (2005). The Mental Health Act was created to give health professionals the power to detain people if they were a danger to themselves or others. The 1983 Act defined mental health as 'mental illness, arrested or incomplete development of mind, psychopathic disorder and any other disorder or disability of the mind'. This was considered overly complex, and the 2007 amendment simply stated mental health as 'any disorder or disability of the mind'. The amendment excludes people with a learning disability provided they are not at risk of self-harm or at risk of harming others.

A 'responsible medical officer' (RMO) usually a consultant psychiatrist, and an approved social worker is required to agree the need to detain for assessment and treatment. However, under the 2007 amendment, this has been widened to include any health professional with an 'approved mental health professional' (AMHP) qualification or responsible clinician (RC) qualification.

The act is written in sections, hence the notion of 'sectioning' people. It gives health professionals the power to assess and treat during the period of detention, and the 2007 amendment allows supervised 'community treatment orders' which can enforce medication if the patient is non-compliant. This is to prevent relapse and hospital admission (the so-called revolving door). Patients have access to an independent mental health capacity advocate (IMCA) whose role is to support the patient and explain their rights under the act.

The Mental Capacity Act (2005) was designed to promote and safeguard patients in decision making by empowering them to make decisions about themselves, and by offering a flexible legal framework which put the patient at the heart of the decision making. It also allows the patient to plan ahead for when they do not have capacity to make decisions (advance directives). The act has five principles which is the legal criteria by which a patient must be assessed and supported.

1. A presumption of capacity: That every adult has the right to make their own decisions and choices and must be assumed to have capacity to do so unless it is proved otherwise.
2. Individuals are supported to make their own decisions: A patient must be given all practicable help before anyone treats them as not being able to make their own decisions.
3. Unwise decisions: the patient must be allowed to make unwise choices.
4. Best interests: Anything done for or on behalf of a patient who lacks mental capacity must be done in their best interests.
5. Less restrictive option: Any decisions made about or for the patient should be done in a way that would interfere less with the person's rights and freedoms of action.

When you are working with a patient who has been assessed by a Best Interest Assessor (BIA) consider the duration of capacity. Someone might not be able to decide immediately, but they may be able to make one at a later date. There should be no presumption that loss of capacity is permanent.

When assessing for capacity the MCA says that patients should be able to do some of the following four things:

1. understand information given to them;
2. retain that information long enough to be able to make the decision;
3. weigh up the information available to make the decision;
4. give their decision.

If the patient is unable to do several of the four things in the list, then 'best interests decision making' should be taken. This should happen taking any advance directive into consideration and in consultation with family, friends, carers and other health professionals. If the patient is judged to lack capacity, an independent mental capacity advocate (IMCA) can make decisions about where the patient lives and any serious medical treatment needed. Read the case study and decide if you think the Best Interest Meeting met the Mr Ellams needs and wishes.

Case Study 7.1: Reginald Ellams

Reginald Ellams is a 70-year-old man with an enduring mental health condition. He lives in a men's hostel and has a shared room on the second floor. Reginald was found unconscious on the bathroom floor. The hostel manager called an ambulance, and Reginald was examined by the paramedics. He was found to be hypothermic, with a weak and irregular heartbeat and breathlessness. He had extensive bruising to his knees.

He was admitted to hospital and blood tests revealed acute renal injury caused by trauma (rhabdomyolysis) possibly from lying on a hard surface for a prolonged period, but also possibly caused by his high dose antipsychotic medication.

Reginald was admitted and warded. Treatment commenced for fluid retention by catheterisation and fluid rehydration via intravenous fluids. Reginald remained confused and had mobility issues.

A best interest meeting was attended by a multidisciplinary team, an AMHP and Reginald's sister to determine the next steps. Although Reginald wanted to return to the hostel, the hostel manager was unable to accommodate him on the ground floor.

The team decided that it was in Reginald's best interests to go to a care home which could offer rehabilitation. This would be a temporary stay for six weeks assessment and reablement. At the end of this period, Reginald would be assessed for mobility and general health as to whether returning to the hostel was feasible.

Activity 7.2   Critical thinking

1. Do you agree with the assessments team's outcome?
2. How do you think the team came to this decision? Use the criteria above and apply it to the case study.

An outline answer is given at the end of this chapter.

A few days after Mr Ellams has been admitted to the care home, his sister received a telephone call from the nurse in charge. She says that Mr Ellams is being a nuisance at night. He is walking along the corridor banging on other resident's doors and shouting he wants to go home. The nurse asks for permission to lock Mr Ellams in his bedroom overnight until the home manager can make an application for Deprivation of Liberty Safeguards (DoLS). The Deprivation of Liberty Safeguards are an amendment to the Mental Capacity Act (2005) and can only be used if the person will be deprived of their liberty in a care home or hospital. The care home manager must ask a local authority if they can have a 'standard authorisation'. Mr Ellams cannot go home, as the hostel cannot accommodate him, but he feels he is being deprived of his liberty.

Mr Ellams' sister agrees he can be locked in overnight for his safety as his mobility is still poor. She insists his community mental health nurse (CPN) is contacted for advice first thing in the morning. Another best interests meeting takes place and Mr Ellams is moved to a secure unit when he can safely move around and access the outdoors when he wishes to. Further information about DOLs is included in the useful web addresses at the end of the chapter.

Childhood emotional and physical trauma

Parenting styles and emotional trauma

Children experience different parenting styles; each has an impact on how successfully the child transitions to adulthood. Diana Blumberg Baumrind (1966) devised original parenting styles and the likely impact on the growing child. The styles are authoritarian (harsh, possibly abusive) permissive (indulgent leading to the 'spoilt' child) and authoritative (firm but responsive).

Affectionless parenting (Bowlby, 1977) is uninvolved or negligent parenting and could be classed as abusive parenting (this is the childhood portrayed in Elton John's biopic *Rocketman*). A childhood lacking warmth, with overly critical parents, leads to children with low self-worth becoming over dependent due to immature emotional development. This has a relationship with neuroticism and suicidal ideation (Goschin et al., 2013).

Differential parenting is gender-based parenting, and considers the styles applied to male and female siblings, formally a traditional upbringing. Siblings have different experiences growing up in the same household, and different personal outcomes in terms of educational opportunity and career prospects. In western societies, this style is considered outdated as it tends to restrict opportunity for females who were socialised to more domestic or caring roles. However, there is a cultural context here as Stewart and Bond (2002) state some south Asian families (Bangladesh and Pakistan) girls are still expected to hold to traditional cultural values.

Erik Erikson (1950) developed the life stage theory, which holds that each developmental stage hinged on how well an individual overcame specific struggles. He suggested that failure to negotiate the struggle could lead to psychological difficulty later in life. Erikson determined that personality was the sum of a person's lifespan experiences. Erikson's great insight was to seat psychological development within societal expectations, hence psycho-social development. Table 7.1 shows the impact of failure to overcome struggles and the likely long-term effect on mental health.

Children and young people's mental health services (CYPMHS) (previously children and adolescent mental health services (CAMHS)) are the NHS and community service providers that offer support for young people experiencing poor mental health. Each area's provision for support varies depending on population demographic and funding availability. This has a relationship with wait times for appointments, which can lead to frustration if provision is patchy. Children with physical ailments or disabilities often also have mental health problems and depression is common. Adolescents coming up to examination periods often experience anxiety and stress which can develop into depression if not promptly recognised and supported.

Children can experience post-traumatic stress disorder if they have suffered physical (and sexual) assaults, domestic violence, traumatic injury (such as a car crash), torture, conflict and war.

Table 7.1   Psychosocial development and the effect on mental health

Trust vs. Mistrust (0–18m)	If the newborn infant's primary carer is inattentive, the child learns the world is inconsistent, resulting in fear
Autonomy vs. Shame (1–3)	The child must learn basic tasks (toileting/eating/dressing) children who are reprimanded for failing will feel shame
Initiative vs. Guilt (3–5)	Children want to explore their world and ask questions, those who are ridiculed will feel guilt
Industry vs. Inferiority (6–11)	Children try to achieve competence in school tasks, ridicule by teachers or friends will lead to withdrawal
Identity vs. Role confusion (12–18)	The child is seeking their own identity, parents who try to force their own vision of the child will lead to identity and role confusion
Intimacy vs. Isolation (18–40)	Failure to develop self esteem can lead to difficulty in sustaining lasting relationships
Generativity vs. Stagnation (40–60)	The feeling of success or failure in life so far, can lead to the 'mid life crisis' feeling that opportunities have been missed/wrong roads taken
Integrity vs. Despair (65+)	Acceptance of life's achievements and disappointments. Failure or guilt can lead to depression and hopelessness

NICE (2018) guidelines support psychological intervention but no longer recommend drug therapy (other than pain relief).

When talking to the parents or carers of children who have witnessed or been involved in traumatic incidents, you should explain the symptoms of post-traumatic stress disorder (PTSD): nightmares, flashbacks, hypervigilance, behavioural difficulties, problems concentrating or/and sleeping, and avoidance of talking about the event. You should point out that, should this continue for more than a month after the event, the child will likely need psychological intervention.

You should note this conversation in the patient's notes for follow up after the child has been discharged.

Access to support may well depend on financial ability, as most psychological support such as counselling is a private (paid for) service. Some types of counselling are offered under 'Improving Access to Psychological Therapy' (IAPT), but this is usually short-term intervention such as cognitive behavioral therapy (CBT), which can be offered for a variety of ailments including depression, anxiety and PTSD.

The first point of call is the school special educational needs coordinator (SENCo) who can offer advice and guidance (signposting) to concerned parents or children. NICE (2019) states:

> In the assessment of a child or young person with depression, healthcare professionals should always ask the patient, and be prepared to give advice, about self-help materials or other methods used or considered potentially helpful by the patient or their parents or carers. This may include educational leaflets, helplines, self-diagnosis tools, peer, social and family support groups, complementary therapies, and faith groups.

Therefore, you should get to know what provision is available within your local clinical commissioning group and your local authority. Quite often, there are partnerships with charities or social enterprise groups, and schools. This complex web of support may be difficult to access unless you or the parents (or caregivers) are persistent.

Anxiety, depression and suicidal ideation

Anxiety is something that we all feel at various times, a sense of nervousness, unease or apprehension about events in our lives. You probably have experienced these things in your life, such as when you were preparing for assessment or starting a new placement. Think about the times you have experienced anxiety; what caused it and how was it resolved?

Activity 7.3   Reflection

Think also about how you experienced anxiety:

Did you worry or over think things?

Did you hear a negative voice in your head?

Did you have difficulty sleeping or sleep too much?

Were you restless, unable to settle?

Not eating properly or eating too much?

Drinking too much alcohol or caffeine drinks?

Did you develop physical symptoms such as a headache, neck ache or back ache?

How did you deal with your anxiety? Did you talk to someone (family, friends, colleagues) or a lecturer or health professional about your worries, or did you keep them to yourself.

Have you learned strategies to support yourself when you are anxious?

As this reflection is based on your own experience of anxiety, there is no outline answer at the end of the chapter.

Feeling anxious is a normal response to situations that cause concern, however, this can develop into something long lasting, such as social anxiety disorder or generalised anxiety disorder (GAD). What causes these disorders to develop is poorly understood, current thinking is that it is part genetics (predisposition) and part environmental, such as trauma, a long-term condition such as epilepsy, arthritis or drug or alcohol misuse. Treatment is usually a combination of anti-anxiolytics such a selective serotonin reuptake inhibitor (SSRIs), or serotonin-norepinephrine reuptake inhibitors (SNRIs) and cognitive behavioural therapy (CBT).

Long-term conditions like anxiety can lead to depression. Depression is quite different from having a low mood or feeling sad. Depression is spectrum of symptoms. Not everyone has all of them but the symptoms impact in some way on daily life. The DSM considers depression to be a psychological reaction to overwhelming emotional or psychological stress. The DSM roughly categorises depression as:

- mild depression: has some impact on daily life;
- moderate depression: has a significant impact on daily life;
- severe depression: nearly impossible to get through day-to-day life.

Depression has both mental and physical symptoms as outlined in Table 7.2.

Table 7.2 Signs and symptoms of depression

Mental	Physical
Continuous sadness or low mood	Speaking slower than usual
Losing interest in things	moving slower than usual
Losing motivation	Aches and pains that cannot be explained
Diminished interest or pleasure in all or most activities	Losing, or gaining weight
Feeling tearful	Constipation
Feeling guilty	Loss of interest in sex
Feeling anxious	Disturbed sleep
Feeling irritable	Loss of energy
Poor concentration	Changes in the menstrual cycle
Finding it hard to make decisions	
Feeling intolerant of other people	
Feeling helpless	
Feeling hopeless	
Low self-esteem	
Feeling worried	
Thinking about suicide	
Thinking about harming yourself	

Source: www.nhsinform.scot/illnesses-and-conditions/mental-health/depression#symptoms-and-causes-of-depression

Activity 7.4   Critical thinking

Examine Table 7.2. Which of these signs and symptoms would you place into the mild, moderate and severe categories?

Compare your answers with the answer given at the end of the chapter.

There is an outline answer at the end of the chapter.

The causes of depression are many, such as post-natal depression caused by hormonal interactions and physical tiredness. The predisposing risk factors in developing depression include long-term stress; military service; being gay, lesbian, bisexual or transgender; physical conditions such as long-term illness (cancer, ME, MS) or neurological disorders, such as stroke and epilepsy; PTSD as a result of trauma (abuse, war, traumatic accidents). Depression also has a relationship with other mental health conditions such as bipolar disorder and schizophrenia.

Depressed people sometimes experience suicidal ideation, passive ideation is wishing you were dead but not actually planning to commit suicide, and active ideation, which is thinking about and planning how to suicide. Suicide is a significant problem in the UK, ONS reports that 11 people per day commit suicide (ONS, 2020b). Women attempt suicide more often than men, but men are more successful in suiciding. Across the UK, the main cause of suicide ideation is money worries and loneliness.

People who have survived a suicide often feel worse after the attempt. Sometimes their family or friends will turn against them, labelling them as selfish or irresponsible. It is important that they receive ongoing support from healthcare professionals to prevent further attempts.

Preventing poor mental health

As discussed earlier, the same socio-economic conditions that impact physical health, also impact mental health. Social and economic disadvantages including racial injustice, discrimination, poverty, unemployment, poor physical health, homelessness, access to drugs and alcohol, and domestic violence are risk factors for developing poor mental health. A public health, community-based approach, based on the principles of advocacy, participation and empowerment, could be funded using a multi-agency model which includes both the public and charitable sectors. This would would involve interventions which target individuals or subgroups of the population who are at significant risk of developing a mental disorder, greater than that of the rest of the population.

Such approaches could include school-based programmes that boost pupil's resilience and self-esteem are health protective and offer good coping strategies that the child can use throughout their life. Workplaces can also offer mental health prevention training to their workforce, along with offering counselling under 'Improving Access to Psychological Therapy' (IAPT). Programmes might be developed that target job seekers to prevent feelings of depression and hopelessness.

Supporting someone with poor mental health

Health promotion with a patient with poor mental health is complex and challenging. Remember that mental and physical health are reciprocal. Patients with cancer, diabetes, heart disease, cardiovascular disease are likely to suffer from anxiety and depression. It is good practice to ask about someone's mental health. Most patients in health and social care settings are likely to have some anxieties, so give them the opportunity to discuss them. Allow your patient free opportunities to talk, use active listening skills as described in Chapter 2. Do not offer advice or opinions. You cannot change what they are going through.

Loneliness is often a cause of poor mental health. Social interactions can prevent your patient from ruminating on their worries. Ask your patient about any hobby or special interest groups they might like to join. Point out that physical activity promotes chemical change in the body by releasing endorphins, running, cycling and dancing are all feel-good mental health promoting activities. Ensure you escalate any concerns and document the conversation.

Learning disability and diagnostic overshadowing

People with a learning disability are more likely to suffer from poor mental health than the general population (mencap.org, 2020). The reasons for this are not settled but likely to include genetic factors related to their learning disability (predisposition), environmental conditions such as poverty, lack of meaningful employment opportunities, abuse, bullying, lack of coping skills, internalised stigma and the effect of discrimination. Poor mental health is not always recognised due to diagnostic overshadowing (see Chapter 2). This is when behaviours are not recognised as poor mental health, but as features of the patient's intellectual or cognitive disability. Some behaviours are considered challenging rather than a nonverbal articulation of mental distress.

Valuing People: A New Strategy for Learning Disability for the 21st Century (2001) and *Valuing People Now* (2004) had a key purpose of 'all people with a learning disability are people first with the right to lead their lives like any other' (mentalhealth.org). A person-centred care process in partnership with the patient. *Valuing People* was subsumed into *Transforming Care* (2015) with varying results, again due to funding deficiencies. The mission statement for *Transforming Care for People with a Learning Disability* is to meet the needs of a complex and diverse groups by tailoring care to their individual needs, central to this is 'Nothing About Us Without Us'.

Care planning and the patient's journey should contain documentation (such as 'My health passport' or 'This is me') which details the patient's preferences in terms of communication strategies, as described in Chapter 2. This is to ensure the patient can give informed consent to treatment.

People with learning disabilities face barriers to access for health screening, dental care, sensory care (Hearing and sight), discharge planning, rehabilitation and suitable accommodation. A multi-disciplinary approach is needed to help the patient navigate and overcome such barriers.

While the number of registered nurses with a learning disability qualification is steadily falling, HEE is working with learning disability service providers to offer dedicated training to nurse associates through the apprenticeship route. Some county councils are offering nurse associates financial inducement to enter the learning disability service sector.

End of life care

Supporting patients through the end of their life is a fact of nursing. There comes a point when we must acknowledge it is time to let the patient go. End of life usually refers to the last year of life and is often used interchangeably with palliative care as a descriptor, although palliative care is about managing symptoms. Approximately half a million people die every year, and nearly all of those deaths will occur within a health or social care setting. End of life care planning involves ensuring the patient lives well and with dignity during their remaining months.

Psychologist Elisabeth Kübler-Ross devised five stages of loss (denial, anger, bargaining, depression and acceptance) these stages are not linear, but cyclical. People who are nearing the end of their lives should be allowed to visit each emotion in their own manner and take as long as they need until they assimilate and accommodate acceptance. While not everyone suffers depression, depression is often unrecognised and undiagnosed in patients nearing the end of life. The main risk factors for depression are diagnosis of a neurodegenerative disorder (Alzheimer's, MS, Parkinson's), poorly managed pain, previous experience of depression and financial distress. Guilt and shame for life events and sadness at things said (and unsaid) or things done (or not done) can also lead to depression.

Medication to treat depression such as selective serotonin reuptake inhibitors (SSRIs) and serotonin-norepinephrine reuptake inhibitors (SNRIs) may take up to four to six weeks to take effect, so their use is limited for those who are within weeks of the end of their life. Psychotherapy should be offered as routine for those nearing the end of their lives, but sadly there is an unacceptable variance in the availability of services and professional expertise available. Most hospices offer such a service but pressure on beds means that many will go without.

Caring for your own mental health

Being a nursing associate demands all your resources, physically, intellectually and emotionally. During the time of the Covid-19 pandemic, nursing associates have cared for patients when they have been exhausted, hungry and thirsty, and have gone above and beyond for their patients. However, so many patients have died from Covid-19 that nursing associates are developing stress-related disorders and their mental health is suffering. Nursing associates working on Covid-19 wards have related their fears for themselves and for their families, fear of catching Covid-19 and taking it home, fear of dying themselves. Many Covid-19 wards had break-out areas for staff when they need a few minutes to gather themselves and access to support for reflection and debriefing (see also Chapter 6).

It is important that you develop health-protecting strategies and know when to call for help. NHS support hubs are being set up which will offer services over the phone with referral to online and one-to-one expert help from qualified mental health clinicians, therapists, recovery workers and psychologists.

1. Grief and sadness

The common symptoms of grief are sadness, anger, tightness in the chest or throat, confusion and insomnia. Each nursing associate will experience grief differently, but some will feel an overwhelming sadness at each life lost.

The Hospice Association have a dedicated telephone line for bereavement support and counselling for health and social care staff 0300 303 4434 (8am–8pm).

2. Anger

In life, we often get angry when we cannot control what is happening to us. When patients die, we sometimes feel anger that we are unable to prevent the death. Anger is related to frustration, and it is important we acknowledge these emotions, so they do not become a problem. It is important that you do not take these feelings home with you and take it out on your family. If you are feeling angry and bewildered, talk to your colleagues and your supervisor about it before you go off duty. Try to go for a run, so you can run off all the anger, running releases endorphins, which should give your mood a boost.

3. Stress and anxiety

It is normal to feel overwhelmed in a crisis, the Covid-19 pandemic began in 2020, and there is every likelihood of the disease continuing to infect the population for some time yet, thus this crisis is going to ebb and flow with the seasons. The danger is that stress will build into anxiety and depression, therefore you need some coping strategies to get you through. The RCN recommends that you use strategies that have worked for you before (RCN, 2020); however, if these strategies include drinking excessive amounts of alcohol, smoking (legal and illegal substances) and overeating, you might need to rethink your strategies for the long haul. Exercising in nature is a great stress buster. When you have free time in daylight hours, take your family for a walk in nature, or to the nearest park. Dance in your kitchen, spend time with your friends and family when possible. Join your local or actual pub for the quiz. You may have essays or assignments to complete but you need down time to recharge your batteries. If you are struggling with assignments, talk to your module leader about extending hand in dates. These are not cast in stone, and you can ask for support when you need it.

Chapter summary

This chapter has introduced you to notions of mental health, and we have explored the legislative framework which governs our work. We examined how mental health is categorised, and the pharmacological and psychological support that is available for treatment options. We also considered the origins of stigma and how it is detrimental to people suffering poor mental health. We looked at some of theoretical perspectives of child mental health and child mental health provision. We also discussed mental health and people with learning disability and the importance of diagnostic overshadowing in their care. Included in this chapter are some health and wellbeing activities you can encourage to promote good mental health, both your patient's and yours.

Activities: brief outline answers

Activity 7.2 Critical thinking (page 130)

The Mental Capacity Act requires someone to take the role of decision maker applying the Best Interest Principle, taking into consideration:

- the specific circumstances and needs of the person;
- the decision that is to be made;
- the urgency of the decision to be made.

1. The AMHP will act as the decision maker, acting in Reginald's best interests, advised by the clinical team and Reginald's sister. The AMHP will Identify all the relevant circumstances. Although Reginald has fluctuating capacity, he has asked to go home (to the hostel), unfortunately his mobility issues preclude this as the hostel cannot accommodate his needs.

2. The AMHP must assess whether the person might regain capacity, as Reginald is expected to regain capacity, normally decision would be delayed until he is able to speak for himself. However, the clinical team have judged him fit for discharge and do not wish to delay transfer to suitable accommodation.

3. Normally an independent mental capacity advocate (IMCA) must be consulted when the decision relates to where the person should live, in this instance the decision was for Reginald to go to a care setting for six weeks assessment. This means that Reginald would receive reablement and the decision postponed until he is capable of making his choice.

Activity 7.4 Critical thinking (page 134)

Table 7.3

Mild	Moderate	Severe
Losing interest in things	Continuous sadness or low mood	Feeling helpless
Losing motivation	Feeling anxious	Feeling hopeless
Diminished interest or pleasure in all or most activities	Feeling irritable	Low self-esteem
Feeling tearful	Poor concentration	Thinking about suicide
Feeling guilty	Finding it hard to make decisions	Thinking about harming yourself
Feeling worried	Feeling intolerant of other people	Disturbed sleep (if prolonged)
Speaking slower than usual	Loss of interest in sex	Changes in the menstrual cycle
moving slower than usual	Loss of energy	
Losing, or gaining weight		
Constipation		

Further reading

The Handbook of Person-Centred Therapy and Mental Health: Theory, Research and Practice (Person-Centred Psychopathology) by Stephen Joseph is a good read to deepen your understanding of the application of person-centred care in mental health.

Man Down: A Guide for Men on Mental Health by Charlie Hoare offers explanations on stigma around male mental health. It is not written for the health practitioner but does offer good advice which is applicable in your practice.

Mental Health and Wellbeing in the Workplace: A Practical Guide for Employers and Employees by Hassan, G. and Butler, D. This book offers expert guidance for improving mental health and supporting those experiencing mental ill health.

Useful websites

A selection of websites which give knowledge and information about mental health, the Mental Capacity Act and mental wellbeing:

www.mind.org.uk/

www.nice.org.uk/guidance/lifestyle-and-wellbeing/mental-health-and-wellbeing

www.proceduresonline.com/resources/mentalcapacity/p_best_interest.html#1.-the-best-interests-principle

www.rcn.org.uk/get-help/member-support-services/counselling-service/Covid-19-and-your-mental-wellbeing

www.samaritans.org/how-we-can-help/if-youre-worried-about-someone-else/supporting-someone-suicidal-thoughts/creating-safety-plan/

www.scie.org.uk/mca/dols

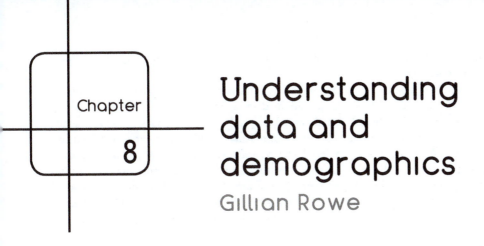

Chapter 8

Understanding data and demographics

Gillian Rowe

Chapter aims

After reading this chapter, you will be able to:

1.   understand the principles of epidemiology;
2.   examine what demography and population means;
3.   identify why health screening is essential to public health;
4.   consider how genomics could revolutionise public health;
5.   investigate the use of digital technology in health promotion.

Introduction

Public health is the science and art of promoting and protecting health and well-being, preventing ill-health and prolonging life through the organised efforts of society.

(Winslow, 1923)

So why is public health a science and why is it an art? By the end of this chapter, you will know the answer to this question.

The plague pandemics were caused by a specific type of flea carrying the Yersinia pestis bacterium. The fleas, carried by black rats, spread the disease from the Mongol heartlands along the silk road to the Black Sea ports and from there to Europe. As a novel zoonotic (zoonotic means diseases that have jumped from animals to humans) disease, it killed up to half of the world's global population several times, the first being the 'Plague of Justinian' in AD 541–750. The plague pandemic came to Europe in the late thirteenth century and early fourteenth century, killing half of the UK population and changing the social structure of society. It became an occasional epidemic in Europe (1665–1666 in London) but devastated China and India in 1855, when 10 million people died. It is now **endemic** in some parts of the world (Saharan Africa, Madagascar and southwestern USA).

AIDs/HIV was described as a 'gay plague' when it arose in 1966. Another zoonotic disease, it spread from Africa to the west. It is still a pandemic on the African continent and has killed approximately 32 million people. Other diseases which have caused pandemics are cholera, smallpox, measles and influenza. First described by Hippocrates in 412 BC, influenza pandemics occur approximately every 30 years.

There have been various influenza pandemics in the twentieth century, such as the so-called 'Spanish flu' of 1918, in which 500 million people were infected and 50 million died. This was an avian H1N1 influenza virus. Further Influenza pandemics included H2N2 influenza virus in 1957–1958 and H3N2 influenza virus in 1968. In 2009, 'swine flu' H1N1pdm09 killed 151,700 people worldwide (CDC estimate). Corona Virus SARs-CoV-2 is the first pandemic of the twenty-first century. Detected in China, it has now spread globally. As of May 2021, it has killed well over three million people worldwide (WHO, 2021c).

Table 8.1   Glossary of terms

Carrier	A person or animal without apparent disease that harbours a specific infectious agent and can transmit the agent to others
Epidemic	Sudden increase in the number of cases of a disease above what is normally expected in that population in that area
Endemic	A disease which is commonly found within populations (e.g., measles, seasonal influenza)
Epidemiology	The study of the distribution and determinants of health-related states or events in specified populations
Frequency	The number of cases of a health event in a defined population, this allows a comparison with the general population
Health indicator	A measure that indicates the state of health of people in a defined population, e.g., the infant mortality rate
Host	A person or other living organism that can be infected by an infectious agent
Outbreak	The same definition for epidemic but within a confined geographical area
Pandemic	A global outbreak of disease
Pattern	The occurrence of health-related events by time, place, and person
Prevalence	is a measure of disease frequency at a point in time
Primary prevention	A public health measure to prevent disease occurrence
Public health	Is concerned with the protection and promotion of the health of people and communities

Reservoir	The habitat in which an infectious agent lives, grows, and multiplies. This includes human, animal, and environmental reservoirs
Screening	The testing of asymptomatic people to determine their likelihood of having a particular disease
Surveillance	The systematic collection, analysis and interpretation of health data
Transmission	The mechanism that an infectious agent is spread. This can be direct or indirect
Vector	An agent that carries and transmits a disease (Tsetse fly is the vector that transmits sleeping sickness)
Zoonosis	An infectious disease that is transmissible from animals to humans

Public health policy frameworks

Health policy concerns plans and actions that are carried out to achieve specific healthcare goals within the UK. Each policy establishes target to be achieved and a roadmap of events to achieve the target. The five core pillars of public health are:

1. behavioural science and health education;
2. biostatistics;
3. environmental health;
4. epidemiology;
5. health services administration.

Public health policy goals for improving the UK population's health are directed at the social determinants of health, including income, education, employment, housing and healthcare services. The UK government (the four nations) have a joint commitment for policy formation to improve the nation's health.

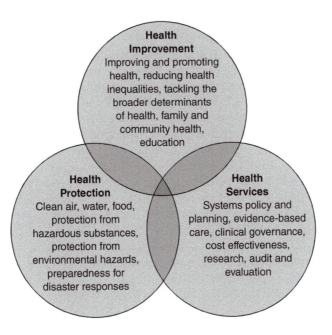

Figure 8.1 The domains of public health

Public Health England (PHE) was formed in 2013, with a mission statement 'to protect and improve the nation's health and wellbeing and reduce health inequalities'. PHE had operational autonomy from the Department of Health and Social Care (DHSC). PHE provided specialist health protection, epidemiology and microbiology services across England. Public Health Scotland, Public Health Wales and PHA Northern Ireland provided similar services to the devolved nations. The PHE was superseded in April 2021 by a new UK wide Health Security Agency (UKHSA) (formerly National Institute for Health Protection (NIHP)). This will combine some of the activities of PHE, the Joint Biosecurity Centre, and the 'Track and Trace service' currently provided by Serco and associates. This new agency will focus on pandemic prevention, health protection and infectious disease management functions. The formation of the UKHSA essentially transfers PHE's health improvement functions back to the DHSC.

Activity 8.1   Critical thinking

The social context of public health examines socio-economic, behavioural and cultural influences.

What do you think these are? Write a list of what you think these influences are.

Compare your answers with the list at the end of the chapter and research any you missed out.

Health inequality

The King's Fund states that 'Health inequalities are avoidable, unfair and systematic differences in health between different groups of people' (kingsfund.org, 2021). Health inequality can mean different things, it can mean health status in communities (such as life expectancy or prevalence of ailments in geographic, demographic and marginalised groups). It can mean access to healthcare provision (such as closure of pharmacies, lack of late-night provision or certain treatments). It can also mean access to affordable housing, secure jobs and clean air.

There is a close relationship between deprivation and life expectancy. Those in the richest areas live approximately seven years longer than those in the poorest areas (known as the Marmot curve). There is a geographical implication with the deprived northern areas having a lower life expectancy than the wealthier south. These figures are replicated in disability-free years. Long-term conditions being an indicator for quality of life and life expectancy.

These figures are not generalisable across all ethnicities. For instance, Gypsy, Roma and Traveller (GRT) communities experience a life expectancy of minus 20 to 28 years compared with settled populations. The GRT community also has greater child mortality and reduced take-up of vaccinations. As this group is socially excluded, they have multiple barriers to access to healthcare, which includes inability to register with a GP surgery or dental clinic. The GRT community face prejudice and discrimination by all sectors of society and as a result are poorly educated and face communication, language and cultural issues. They are often quite fearful of contact with health professionals based on historical institutional abuses.

The intersections between quality of life, life expectancy and deprivation are noticeably clear. These were originally highlighted in the 1980 Black Report and supported by further research by Michael Marmot (Marmot Review 2008, 2018) which identified that people experience systematic, unfair and avoidable differences in their health. Both the NHS Five Year Forward View and the NHS Long-Term Plan made prevention a priority.

Primary, secondary and tertiary healthcare provision

- Primary healthcare: the first level of contact between individuals and families with the health system, primary healthcare is to serve the community. It includes care for mother and child, such as family planning, immunisation, treatment of common diseases or injuries, provision of essential facilities and health education. This would include GPs, district nurses, opticians, dentists, pharmacy, health centre provision.
- Secondary healthcare: a patient who has been provided with primary care may be referred to a secondary care professional – a specialist with expertise on the patient's issue. These are consultant-led services, which include psychology, psychiatry and orthopaedics. Secondary care is usually (but not always) delivered in a hospital/clinic with the initial referral being made by the primary care professional.
- Tertiary healthcare: once a patient is hospitalised, they may require highly specialised treatment and care within the hospital. Tertiary care requires professionals, usually surgeons, with specific expertise in each field, to carry out investigation and treatment for the patient. Examples include neurosurgery, cardiac surgery and cancer management.

Primary, secondary and tertiary public health

1. Primary prevention aims to prevent disease or injury before it occurs. This is done by preventing exposures to hazards that cause disease or injury. Altering unhealthy or unsafe behaviours and environments that can lead to disease or injury and increasing resistance to disease or injury should exposure occur. For example, legislation and enforcement to ban or control the use of hazardous products such as asbestos, or to mandate safe and healthy practices, such as use of seatbelts. Education about healthy and safe habits which would include eating well, smoking cessation and exercising regularly.

   Primary public health prevention also includes childhood and adult immunisation against infectious diseases. Implementing food safety legislation at the local level, and the oversight of water companies who provide sewerage and piped clean water supplies. This comes under the heading of communicable disease outbreak management. Working with public health organisations is the Health and Safety Executive which monitors reporting systems such as Reporting Infectious Diseases and Dangerous Occurrences Regulations (RIDDOR 2013) and Control of Substances Hazardous to Health (COSHH)

2. Secondary prevention aims to reduce the impact of a disease or injury that has already occurred. Such as encouraging personal strategies to prevent re-injury or recurrence. Implementing programmes to return people to their original health and function to prevent long-term problems. This would include diet and exercise programmes to prevent further heart attacks or strokes, and NHS screening tests and regular examinations to detect disease in its earliest stages (for example, mammograms to detect breast cancer).

   Tertiary prevention aims to soften the impact of an ongoing illness or injury that has lasting effects. This is done by helping people manage long-term, often-complex health problems and injuries. This is done by supporting individuals and groups with cardiac or stroke rehabilitation programmes or chronic disease management programmes (diabetes, arthritis, depression) these support groups encourage members to share strategies for living well.

Public health data

The government green paper 'Advancing our health: prevention in the 2020s' obliges making effective use of data and technology a central theme. Primary data on health is collated from information provided by primary healthcare providers GP surgeries, clinics, dentists, pharmacies and secondary providers, such as hospital admissions. Data is also collected from death certificates. This data offers a broad base of knowledge which can be interrogated further. Data can also be collected from health surveys such as the School's Survey (see below) which charts tobacco and alcohol use. There are many longitudinal studies, such as the Millennium Cohort Study, which follows children born in 2000 and charts their social and economic conditions, as well as their health (advantages and disadvantages), or the National Child Development Study, which began in 1958 with the aim of achieving an improved understanding of the factors affecting human development over the whole lifespan.

The ten-yearly national census, currently hosted by the Office for National Statistics (ONS) has been undertaken since 1801. The census includes questions on physical and mental health, long-term conditions and disability. This data capture informs government health services planning both locally and nationally.

Data collected for health purposes can be used for administrative, legal, political or economic purposes such as using health surveys and comparing with sales of tobacco products or alcohol or to determine the effectiveness of anti-tobacco and alcohol initiatives. Data collection on the environment, such as air and water quality (drinking and bathing), availability of homes, green-space recreation opportunities and access to jobs all contribute to understanding of health in populations. Other environmental monitoring includes adherence to health and safety at work legislation and food safety.

In the UK, there are 35 notifiable infectious diseases (NOIDS). The diagnosing clinician is required to inform the Public Health Agency of such diseases as tuberculosis, meningitis, E. coli, campylobacter and salmonella. The 'yellow card' system is the reporting of side effects (adverse drug reactions) from medications or vaccines, hosted by the Medicines and Healthcare Products Regulatory Agency (MHRA). The agency collects information and monitors medicines safety concerns. It also covers medical devices such as implants, infusion pumps and scanners. Some further diseases are reportable to the World Health Organization (WHO) such as cholera, plague and yellow fever.

Evidence-based public health

Brownson et al. (2017) consider evidence-based public health practice to be 'the development, implementation, and evaluation of effective programmes and policies in public health' they consider the application of systematic use of data and information systems to programme models of behaviour. We should ask if the interventions are founded on established scientific studies and if there are any lessons to be learned for both successful and unsuccessful interventions, and if those can interventions be applied across settings.

Evaluating interventions requires interpretation of the scientific literature and systematic reviews. Decisions are made based on the best available peer-reviewed evidence (both quantitative and qualitative). Applying programme planning frameworks (based on health behaviour theory), conducting sound evaluation and disseminating what is learned. Earlier in this chapter we examined the primary, secondary and tertiary principles of public health. The fourth, or quaternary, principle is protection from harmful medical intervention. This is defined by Jamoulle and Roland (1995) as 'action taken to identify a patient or a population at risk of over-medicalization, to protect them from invasive medical interventions and provide for them care procedures which are ethically acceptable'. This means that assurances should be given to individuals and populations that health planning should use evidence-based decision making to evaluate any intervention before it is widely disseminated.

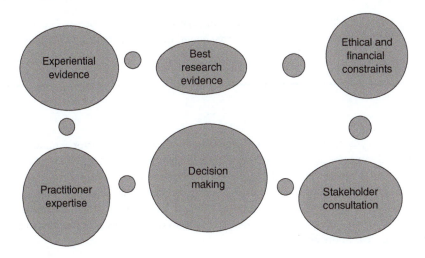

Figure 8.2   Evidence-based decision making

(Source: WGO.org)

An example of evidence-based decision making is the School's Survey, which seeks to determine at what age children begin to use tobacco, drugs and alcohol in order to tailor interventions. The research is carried out by Ipsos MORI for the NHS and shared with various government departments.

Case study 8.1: Smoking, drinking and drug use among young people in England

Smoking, drinking and drug use among the young: School's Survey. These are some of the issues asked about to determine the prevalence of smoking, drinking and drug taking among school children:

- the number of pupils who have never smoked, drunk alcohol or taken drugs;
- the age at which pupils tried tobacco, alcohol or drugs;
- types of alcohol and drugs taken;
- how often pupils smoke, drink and take drugs;
- e-cigarette use;
- where pupils obtain cigarettes, alcoholic drinks and drugs.

The purpose of the survey is to determine predictors of the likelihood of smoking, drinking and drug use among schoolchildren, and extrapolate likely lifetime use. The government's Public Health harm reduction plan is to reduce the number of young people smoking by 3 per cent by 2022.

Activity 8.2 Critical thinking

What do you think the 'Smoking, drinking and drug use among young people in England' survey tells you and do you think there is anything that could impact negatively on this survey?

An outline answer is given at the end of the chapter.

The School's Survey is used to inform public health planning and education. Smoking, drinking and drug use amongst young people are key public health concerns. It will inform public health practitioners at which age anti-smoking, alcohol and drug messages should begin in schools and on media. The data is used by central and local government to better understand why these behaviours occur so new initiatives can be developed. The survey also determines who has influenced habit uptake (friends, family, peers, social media) and allow programmes to be devised to counteract these influences.

Public health and epidemiology

Epidemiology is the scientific study of health and health-related events in defined populations. It considers the social determinants of health and the frequency and distribution of diseases. Epidemiology is data driven, which means it relies on a systematic collection of data for analysis and interpretation. The science of epidemiology includes information from other research fields, such as biostatistics and informatics, and biologic, economic, social and behavioural science.

Epidemiology as a science was first described by Hippocrates, who made the distinction between an epidemic (a visiting disease such as plague) and endemic (a disease resident in a community such as the common cold). Joaquín de Villalba was the first to use the term epidemiology in 1802 to study epidemics. Modern epidemiology began in London with the work of Jon Snow. He was a doctor from Tyneside who also gave Queen Victoria anaesthesia during childbirth. Snow had already hypothesised that cholera came from drinking infected water, but germ theory was still in its infancy, and cholera was assumed to be the result of a miasma of bad air. Snow knew that cholera affected the digestive system, not the respiratory system, but he had no way of proving his theory.

In 1854, he investigated a cholera outbreak in Soho, between Regent Street and Dean Street. He drew a map of the area and put an X next to each house which had an occupant who died from cholera (see Figure 8.3), from this, he worked out the Broad Street pump was responsible. He persuaded the council to take the handle off the pump, and the outbreak ended. He also proved that cholera was waterborne, something that was not accepted by the medical profession until after Snow's death.

Snow's map is a geographic visualisation of the data recorded in his diaries, which linked disease with location.

Snow was aided in his research by two innovations, one was the establishment of the Post Office; by law, houses had to have a number. The other innovation was the establishment in 1837 of the Register of Births, Marriages, and Deaths, which gave the date and cause of death. It also gave their address. Now Snow had the exact address, date and cause of death. He used this data for his map.

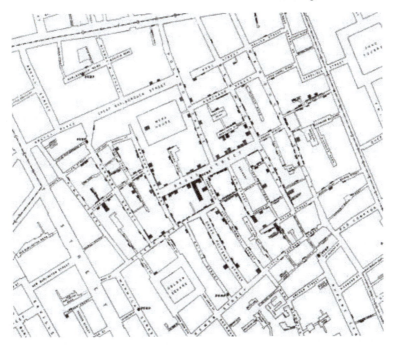

Figure 8.3 Jon Snow's 1854 map

Snow's legacy

Nineteenth-century epidemiology concentrated on infectious diseases, by the twentieth century non-infectious disease was investigated, and, after the Second World War, chronic diseases. In the 1960s epidemiological principles were applied to the eradication of smallpox globally. From the 1980s, violence and injuries at work were added to the research cannon. Emerging threats such as AIDs/HIV, Ebola, legionella, severe acute respiratory syndrome (SARS) and drug-resistant mycobacterium tuberculosis have been investigated, tracked and monitored, informing global governments of public health responses to contain and control disease.

Genomics and public health

Genetics is the study of single genes such as those that cause fragile x disorder or cystic fibrosis. Genomics studies gene combinations or all the genes in a single organism to determine how they interact with each other and how environmental factors can affect an organism's growth and development. Thus, genomic researchers examine how genes interact with environments and lifestyles to cause such diseases as diabetes, cancer and heart disease.

Beginning in the 1990s, molecular and genetic epidemiology is now offering insights into the use of genomics to estimate disease heritability. The mapping of the human genome was the world's largest collaborative biological project, mapping more than three billion nucleotides took 13 years. An international consortium hosted by the American National Institute for Health (NIH) located a mosaic of genes by 2003, leaving knowledge gaps in some chromosomes which are slowly being filled in by further research. In 2007, the first individual to have their entire genome mapped was James Watson. This was fitting since it was his work, along with Francis Crick, Maurice Wilkins and Rosalind Franklin that determined the double helix shape of deoxyribonucleic acid (DNA).

Since the human genotype was first completed, studies have detailed the genetic basis of diseases ranging from inflammatory bowel disease to hypertension, viruses and bacterial infections. Genotyping has allowed the development of biotechnology and biologic medications, and has determined some of the mutations that cause cancer. Genetic technology will help to prevent infectious diseases spreading and enable rapid response and more effective surveillance.

The benefits of genomic research will give us information about how diseases develop, in what circumstances different genetic variations contribute to disease progression. In time, research will establish why some people seem immune to certain diseases and others are not. This should help to develop an understanding for risk prediction in relation to the onset of a specific disease.

Another benefit will be the ability to protect subgroups within populations, such as those with genetic predispositions to sickle cell anaemia and cardiovascular disease (CVD). Medication research does not generalise well to ethnic minorities who have different genetic susceptibilities and inheritance. For example, Chinese men and women seldom develop CVD, whereas people of south Asian origin have the highest rates within the UK. Yet the same people of south Asian origin have low rates of cancer. These genetic mysteries will one day be solved by genomic research.

There are ethical implications within genomic research, for instance genetic screening of newborn babies can identify those at risk of genetic disease. If a child is diagnosed as having or likely to develop a genetic disorder, this has implications for the child, the parents and the wider family. Should the family receive genetic counselling? Indeed, should the parents be restricted to a single child due to associated health costs? Therefore, a conversation about ethics and equity needs to take place before decisions about individuals, subgroups and populations are taken at national level.

Using electronic data

There is a great deal of evidence that proves the major issues facing public health are the social determinants of health such as income, education, housing and clean air. These affect populations and individuals, especially those living in areas of deprivation. Research is now undertaken using electronic health records (EHRs), for example to examine prevalence, frequency, onset, persistence, severity and outcome of childhood asthma. GPs' electronic data can be processed by variable (such as geographic location) and comparisons made for research purposes. Patient reported symptoms or patient-generated health data (PGHD) can be migrated onto GP platforms.

Data captured from mobile devices, such as smartphones, activity trackers and other sensors can be integrated into healthcare systems for real time results. For example, continuous glucose monitoring (CGM) for Type 1 diabetes uses an implanted device to automatically monitor blood sugar levels (see Figure 8.5). Readings are sent to an app on a smart phone and transferred to a clinician and recorded on the EHR. Alerts can be set up if the patient has consistent spikes to seek medical help. An epilepsy tracker is in development, and this will hopefully provide more personalised care for epileptics. Patient arm-worn activity devices which send data to apps can be used by healthcare professionals to monitor fitness activities to combat obesity in children and families. These devices can be incorporated into telemedicine appointments which allows GPs and consultants to 'see' more patients in the working day.

Smart phone apps have been used by Covid-19 victims. Over 4 million people use a symptom tracker to share symptoms with NHS and Kings College university scientists. This allows researchers to identify novel symptoms and disseminate information. The app is evolving over time allowing participants to discover how their data is informing research.

Integrated medical devices are used in surgery and ITU, so the data collected by medical devices is automatically uploaded into the electronic patient record (EPR). Electronic observations can calculate a patient's early warning score. This means that if a patient is deteriorating, alerts inform for rapid response. In day clinics, observations and assessments such as urinalysis, blood pressure or weight can be uploaded before the consultant sees the patient, allowing for a review of notes and clinical test results beforehand.

There are barriers to full integration of smart devices. The first is interoperability as device manufacturers prefer to use their own platforms, however, as the 'internet of things' gathers pace,

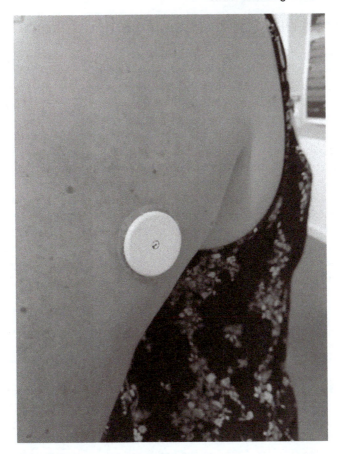

Figure 8.5   Diabetes flash monitor © G. Rowe

open-source software should become more common. The other main barrier is cost. The NHS tends to use older and therefore cheaper technology. Also, the cost of network infrastructure at the bedside is a huge investment, especially for older hospitals which are generally smaller and have less space.

Data legislation

NHS data has its own specific legislation included into the Data Protection Act (DPA) 2018. Article 9 stipulates that the collection and processing of personal data must be fair, lawful and transparent. The EU GDPA legislation states:

> processing data is necessary for the purposes of preventive or occupational medicine, for the assessment of the working capacity of the employee, medical diagnosis, the provision of health or social care or treatment or the management of health or social care systems and services on the basis of Union or Member State law or pursuant to contract with a health professional and subject to conditions and safeguards.

Although the UK has left the EU, this is still current legislation.

Data security is an issue. Protecting e-data from hackers or other security breaches is expensive. Anonymised NHS data is available to researchers, however, individual patients may be offered secure portals to upload and access their data.

Health screening across the life span

Health screening is a public health activity which examines people who are apparently healthy. Different screening is offered to different age groups, pregnant women (hepatitis, HIV, syphilis, sickle cell) and screening for Downs and Patau's disease in the baby. The newborn will be screened for rare conditions by heel prick and tested for hearing and any physical abnormalities.

Young et al. (2018) state that 50 per cent of the population will be diagnosed with cancer in their lifetime. Cervical screening for women begins at 25 and is offered every three years until age 64. There is some public pressure to reduce the age to 20, following some well publicised cases of early death from cervical cancer that could have been picked up if testing commenced earlier.

Breast screening begins at age 50 to 70 for women. All adults aged 65 and over are offered bowel screening, and abdominal aortic aneurysm (AAA) screening is targeted mainly at men, but women can ask for a scan too. Young et al. (2018) state that screening uptake 'for breast, cervical and colorectal cancer have uptake rates of 71 per cent, 73 per cent and 52 per cent'. Encouraging uptake is therefore a key public health strategy. People over 65 are offered a pneumonia vaccine and over 70s are offered a Shingles vaccine; both vaccinations are given once only and can be given at any time of the year.

Let us examine the case study on bowel cancer screening. As you can see, the uptake is far lower than other types of screening.

Case study 8.2: Bowel cancer screening

The uptake of bowel cancer screening was poor. Less than 50 per cent of those invited to screen participated. There were several reasons for this. The Faecal Occult Blood test (gFOBT) required the participant to wipe several samples of faeces with a spatula. This meant catching stool samples in a container and then disposing of the contents. This test was replaced in 2019 with the Faecal Immunochemical Test (FIT) which requires only one sample and has a greater uptake (52 per cent).

The barriers to uptake include those with religious objections, those with physical disabilities, those with sensory (eyesight) loss and those with learning disabilities. Fear of a positive diagnosis was often cited reason for refusal to participate. Men from all backgrounds were also reluctant to participate.

Activity 8.3   Critical thinking

You are working at a GP surgery which offers a five-yearly NHS check-up for men. You are asked to contribute in encouraging people to participate in bowel screening. What things could you say?

An outline answer is given at the end of the chapter.

Researchers considered what barriers there are to male participation in bowel screening and what public health promotion strategies could be used to encourage uptake. Men are significantly more likely to develop bowel cancer, so screening is health promoting. The question was turned around, and researchers asked, 'why are women more likely to participate in screening?' Findings identified that women were comfortable with contact with health professionals. They are positively engaged with their own wellbeing, having already participated in cervical and breast screening by the time they reached bowel screening age. The success of the 'Movember' movement, which encouraged men to grow a moustache in November, as part of testicular and prostate cancer awareness led to the 'Decembeard' campaign, run by the charity Bowel Cancer UK, to encourage men to grow a beard to highlight bowel cancer awareness.

Vaccine data and evidence-based public health

Immunisation uptake is still suffering from the impact of Andrew Wakefield's 1998 corrupt research. Wakefield alleged that there was a link between the measles, mumps and rubella (MMR) vaccine and autism. However, over 100 research groups have failed to reproduce Wakefield's study, and it later emerged that Wakefield had a financial incentive in making the association. The resulting outbreaks of preventable diseases in so called 'Wakefield cohorts' is still high. In 2019, there were 5,042 laboratory confirmed cases of mumps (Kmietowicz, 2020). Mumps (Parotitis) is a contagious viral infection spread by droplets and kissing. Most cases of mumps occur in people between 17 and 34 years of age who have not received two doses of the MMR vaccine. Occasionally, mumps can lead to viral meningitis if the virus moves into the outer layer of the brain, and sterility in men if the testicles are inflamed. Rarely, some people experience hearing loss or become deaf.

Parents are still refusing vaccination for their children, despite the overwhelming evidence in favour of the vaccine and an extensive public health campaign. Public health research indicates vaccine hesitancy may be a result of complacency due to the perception that there is a low risk of contagion and the rise of the anti-vax movement on social media.

Some locales have particularly low take up of the MMR, such as Leeds, which had 89 per cent of children immunised. In order to achieve herd immunity a vaccination rate of 95 per cent is required. We are all familiar with the R (reproduction) rate for Covid-19 and the need to keep it below one. The R rate for measles in Leeds is currently 14 (Cooper, 2021). Many cases of MMR are in young adults who did not have the vaccine post-Wakefield. They are catching the diseases at university, music festivals and other large public events. This led to the World Health Organization removing the UK's measles-free status.

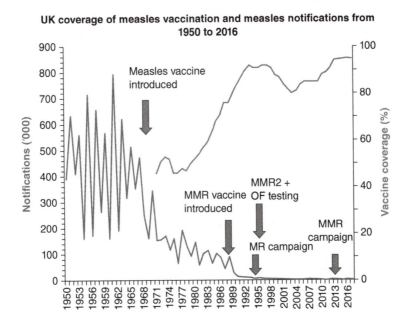

UK coverage of measles vaccination and measles notifications from 1950 to 2016

Figure 8.6 Measles PHE

Activity 8.4   Critical thinking

Examine the chart showing measles vaccination and notification from 1950 to 2016, think about the following and jot your thoughts down.

- Identify the impact of the vaccine on the number of notifications.
- Look at the evidence after the MMR vaccine was introduced, what happened?
- Examine the vaccination line at the end of the 1980s to 2001, What do you think might have caused the reduction in uptake?
- How effective were the two public health campaigns?

Compare your thoughts with answers given at the end of the chapter.

The perception that it is better for the child to catch measles rather than have the vaccination is an erroneous one. The nonspecific immune system uses engulfing cells called phagocytes; these are cells that eat invading organisms (think Pacman). These are the link between the nonspecific and specific immune system. Once a phagocyte has engulfed the infectious agent, it acts as an antigen presenting cell, which then stimulates the mediated system. The mediated system white cells make T lymphocytes antibodies which fight a specific disease. T lymphocytes are capable of remembering the infective agent and can reproduce at a rate of 2,000 antibody molecules per second when required.

Unfortunately, measles destroys all the T lymphocytes that hold immune memory, extinguishing immunity to diseases. This leaves the individual susceptible to other infections, including those previously experienced or vaccinated against. Research by Mina et al. (2015) demonstrated it can take up to three years for the immune system to recover, and this has an impact on child mortality.

Immunisation

Babies are immunised at 8 weeks (6-in-1), 12 weeks (6-in-1 second dose), 16 weeks (6-in-1 third dose) and at 12 months (MMR, Hib/MenC vaccine fourth dose, PCV second dose). All these vaccinations provoke an immune response, so it is not uncommon for the baby to be a bit feverish for a day or two after the vaccination. Unfortunately, this can put some parents off further vaccinations because they do not understand the side effects of vaccines. Therefore, it is important to explain to parents that their baby's immune system is working when they are feverish, and this is a desired result. Children receive a preschool booster, a 3-in-1 teenage booster and the HPV vaccination at 12 years and a booster a year later. The MenACWY vaccine is offered in the final year at school and at freshers' events at university to prevent meningitis and septicaemia.

Using digital technology to promote healthy lifestyles

Public health messages using social media have had a problematic past as the messages were perceived as paternalistic and, frankly, dull. NHS digital campaigns have been revitalised and now provide a visually attractive informative site under the NHS website and 'Change4Life' platform. However, public health has been slow to recognise that internet searches for health information has left the public at the mercy of the commercial sector and charlatans. There is a whole ecosystem of misinformation, disinformation and quackery that promotes health conspiracy theories to the detriment of legitimate health promotion.

This was witnessed most clearly in 2020 when anti-vax and anti-mask groups attracted large followings and public protest demonstrations. It would be easy to dismiss these groups as health denying, but social psychologists who have explored this phenomenon suggested that anti-vax and anti-maskers do not believe there is a pandemic, therefore vaccination and mask wearing is not necessary. There are some conspiracy theorists who believe the threat of Covid-19 has been exaggerated by the government to control the populace. Psychological reactance explains that when people feel threatened, they will offer counter arguments or explanations in order to reassert their autonomy and capacity for choice, and will become angry when challenged. This is also an explanation for health promotion resistance.

Research in America by Professor Abrams (2020) showed that young people perceived themselves to be at little risk of Covid-19, and therefore do not view their behaviour as risk taking. Abrams also makes the valid point that humans use nonverbal communication and mask wearing acts as a barrier to reading facial expressions, so there is an inherent dislike of masks. There is a strong tribal and political divide in anti-mask conspiracy organisations. In and out group theory (Tajfel et al., 1979) explains the reinforcers of public health versus individual personal freedom approaches. This phenomenon was also seen in San Francisco in 1918, during the 'Spanish flu' pandemic, when an anti-mask league was formed, stating that mask wearing was contrary to civil liberties. Recent anecdotal evidence (Taylor and Asmundson, 2021) suggests that the mixed messages given out by both the World Health Organization and the UK government on the effectiveness of mask wearing has had an impact on public compliance. It is clear that any public health messaging needs to be consistent and unambiguous for it to be effective.

NHSX and NHS improvement have various digital health programmes trialling, however, due to the pandemic 'NHS@home' has been expanded in terms of provision and speed of roll out. Patients who would normally attend hospital clinic appointments to monitor their health conditions have been given the opportunity to attend 'virtual wards'. For example, home-based spirometry has been offered to patients with cystic fibrosis. This was commenced as 'project breathe', a research-based data collection activity to understand whether measuring things like lung function, oxygen levels, activity and weight at home can reduce the number of hospital appointments for people with CF (Allen, 2021). The pulse oximetry programme was expanded and rapidly rolled out to support the recovery of those with Covid-19-related respiratory issues. The readings were linked to app-based check-ins with clinicians, who monitored their condition in real time and could offer advice if a patient were deteriorating (nhs@home, 2021).

Public Health England were concerned with the effects of lockdown on weight and morale. In response, they devised a digital challenge called 'couch to 5k'. Data capture shows that over a million people downloaded the phone app fitness tool. Research (see Chapter 6) by Rychter et al. (2020) demonstrated the link between obesity and Covid-19 mortality rate, so the app was designed for use by people with poor fitness levels, to encourage them to take positive steps for their health and fitness.

Using MECC to influence health behaviours

Examination of the chart 'factors influencing health' shows that behavioural factors have significant impact in health and wellbeing and that mitigating behaviour is the goal of health promotion. The Prevention and Lifestyle Behaviour Change Competence Framework has been developed to guide healthcare professionals in the art of health promotion by using good practice methodologies. The framework offers core competences for nurse associates to deliver techniques and approaches to support individuals to change lifestyle and behaviours detrimental to health.

The Positive Behavioural Support Framework (2015) offers a theoretical and evidence base which supports those with challenging behaviours. The framework is a practical guide for supporting individuals with an intellectual or cognitive disability and focuses on matching support needs with capability. It offers a person-centred plan mitigating challenging behaviour while allowing the individual to achieve meaningful choices and aspirations, using a least restrictive approach. It is important that you understand your patient's communication preferences and have strategies to prevent miscommunication or diagnostic overshadowing.

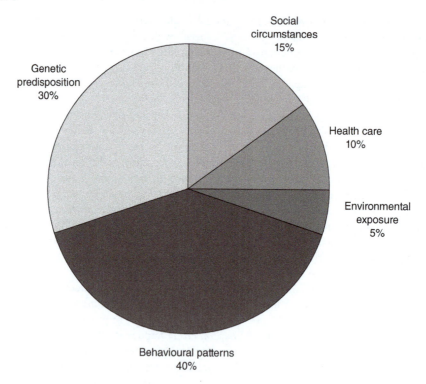

Figure 8.4 Factors influencing health

Nursing associates should always be alert to opportunities for brief conversations offering advice using making every contact count (MECC) and be able to explore an individual's views about their lifestyle and behaviours. This needs to be conducted in a sensitive non-judgemental manner. There is an art to MECC conversations, by being open, friendly and engaging, using positive body language in a manner that encourages the individual to feel comfortable talking to you. Earlier in this chapter, we considered how people use psychological defence mechanisms to reject unwelcome information, so be prepared to offer knowledgeable counter arguments and signpost to people or organisations who can help them to achieve their goals.

- Understand that people may not have the same level of education that you do, so do not assume they will comprehend you if you use technical jargon. Keep your language simple.
- They may also have different religious, cultural and personal beliefs, and you should acknowledge them when offering choice making.
- You should also talk about the individual's circumstances and how these can affect healthy choice making, offering advice about services that are beyond the person's financial research is counterproductive.
- Encourage the individual to talk about their general health and any wellbeing concerns and ask them to assess how risk-taking behaviours are impacting on their mental and physical health.
- Ask what would motivate them to change their behaviour. This gives the individual a sense of ownership and autonomy.

- Ask about barriers to making healthy changes, and how they can be overcome, offer a menu of alternatives which support their success in making healthy changes.
- Always value any success and reinforce this with a positive message when they have not achieved as much as they had hoped to.

Chapter summary

This chapter has examined public health and public health policy areas. We then discussed the collection of data and how it is used to inform health policies and agencies. We considered the genomic revolution applicability to public health and then examined the use of electronic data and its use across the health provision spectrum. We discussed health screening services and looked at uptake and considered ways that uptake could be improved. We went on review digital media and social media and deliberated on the effectiveness of digital campaigns. We talked about immunisation and considered the legacy causes of low vaccine uptake and the implications for herd immunity. We answered the question posed at the beginning of the chapter – what is the science and the art of public health? – the science being the understanding, interpretation and application of data and the art being using communication skills to make improvements to health and wellbeing.

Activities: brief outline answers

Activity 8.1 Critical thinking (page 144)

list of socio-economic, behavioural, and cultural influences

How many of these did you get?

• Social networks	• Access to services and amenities
• Family background	• Geographical area
• Social class	• Housing
• Culture	• Economic/employment status
• Media	• Nutritional Status
• Ethnicity	• Drug and Alcohol Abuse
• Education	• Sexual behaviour
• Truancy and Bullying	
• Wealth	

Activity 8.2 Critical thinking (page 148)

Smoking, drinking and drug use among the young: School's Survey.

What does this survey tell us?

This research indicates how pupils smoke or take drugs and alcohol and what age they start using. This gives a strong indication of when interventions should be put in place in schools to prevent tobacco/drugs/alcohol use.

The negatives are that it presumes the pupils are telling the truth, they might lie about substance use either saying they do use substances (when they do not) or saying they do not use substances (when they do).

The survey does not include questions on access to pornography or obesity questions when this information could be collected at the same time.

Activity 8.3 Critical thinking (page 152)

Bowel Cancer Screening: People trust nurses and clinicians so a short conversation could reinforce the importance of screening. As many people resist screening because they are fearful of the result, you could give reassurance that early intervention reduces the chance of dying from bowel cancer. If polyps are found they may develop into cancer over time, so removing polyps during a colonoscopy can reduce the chances of developing bowel cancer in the future.

Activity 8.4 Critical thinking (page 154)

As you can see, measles is endemic in the population at 1950 and the notification fluctuates (epidemics) between 180,000 and 800,000 prior to the introduction of the vaccine in 1965, when numbers fall significantly.

Once the MMR is introduced, the spikes disappear, measles epidemics no longer routinely occur.

The vaccination line shows the impact of Wakefield's corrupt study which was reported widely and disseminated throughout the UK media. Parents were refusing vaccination and measles spiked again.

It is clear that the first campaign was less successful, however, both public health campaigns together evidenced success in increasing vaccinations from 2004 onward, but vaccination has stabilised at about 90 per cent from 2017–2020 (Nuffield trust.org, 2021), the WHO requirement for measles-free status is 95 per cent.

Further reading

Brownson, R., Baker, T. Deshpande. A, Gillespie, K. (2017) *Evidence-based Public Health.* Oxford: Oxford University Press. This is a useful, professionally written, easy-to-read introduction to evidence-based public health.

Tajfel, H., Turner, J., Austin, W. and Worchel, S. (1979) *An Integrative Theory of Intergroup Conflict. Organizational Identity: A Reader.* Monterey, CA: Brooks and Cole. This is a seminal text for understanding group behaviour and the factors that influence group behaviours. It could be read alongside Becker, H. (2018) *Outsiders: Studies in the Sociology of Deviance,* which explains notions of deviant behaviour.

Useful websites

ukdataservice.ac.uk/get-data/key-data/cohort-and-longitudinal-studies

The UK data service collection includes major UK government-sponsored surveys, cross-national surveys, longitudinal studies, UK census data and is freely available to students, researchers and academics.

www.england.nhs.uk/wp-content/uploads/2018/04/social-media-policy.pdf

Social media and attributed digital content policy should be read before posting any content to social media in a professional capacity in order to protect yourself and your employers.

www.england.nhs.uk/6cs/wp-content/uploads/sites/25/2015/05/pbs-comp-framework.pdf

The positive behavioural support framework is aimed at mitigating challenging behaviour, but its values should be available for all individuals who you work with.digital.nhs.uk/

NHS Digital has a huge website which covers such things as NHS cybersecurity, statistics and reports, making connections between the NHS and partner organisations and offering health information to the general public.

Glossary

Endemic A disease which is commonly found within populations (e.g., measles, seasonal influenza)

Epidemic Sudden increase in the number of cases of a disease above what is normally expected in that population in that area

Epidemiology The study of the distribution and determinants of health-related states or events in specified populations

Frequency The number of cases of a health event in a defined population, this allows a comparison with the general population

Habitus Bourdieu's theory of internalised structures, schemes of perception and action common to all members of the same group or class

Host A person or other living organism that can be infected by an infectious agent

MECC Making every contact count, short interventions offering advice and signposting assistance

Obesogenic environment the role environmental factors play in determining both nutrition and physical activity

Outbreak The same definition for epidemic but within a confined geographical area

Pandemic A global outbreak of disease

Prevalence A measure of disease frequency at a point in time

Primary prevention A public health measure to prevent disease occurrence

Public health Concern with the protection and promotion of the health of people and communities

Reflect back repeating what the patient has told you, in order to confirm an understanding of what is being said

Reservoir The habitat in which an infectious agent lives, grows and multiplies. This includes human, animal and environmental reservoirs

Salutinogenic Antonovsky's theory which is a positive health model that is concerned with the relationship between health, stress and coping

Screening The testing of asymptomatic people to determine their likelihood of having a particular disease

Self-belief confidence in your own abilities or judgment

Glossary

Social reflexivity   Anthony Giddens theory that we have the ability to change identity in the light of new information

Surveillance   The systematic collection, analysis and interpretation of health data

Transmission   The mechanism that an infectious agent is spread. This can be direct or indirect

Zoonosis   An infectious disease that is transmissible from animals to humans

References

Abrams, D. (2020) *The Psychology behind Adherence to Mask Policies*. Available at: www.aamc.org/news-insights/science-and-psychology-behind-masking-prevent-spread-Covid-19

Action for Children (2017) *Action for Children: It Starts with Hello Report*. Available at: www.actionforchildren.org.uk/media-centre/

Akkilinc, F. (2019) The body language of culture. *International Journal for Innovation Education and Research*, 7: 32–9. doi: 10.31686/ijier.Vol7.Iss8.1639. Available at: www.researchgate.net/publication/335689301_The_Body_Language_of_Culture

Allen, J. (2021) *Cystic Fibrosis Trust*. Available at: www.cysticfibrosis.org.uk/get-involved/clinical-trials

Allen, M. (2014) *Local Action on Health Inequalities: Building Children and Young People's Resilience in Schools*. Institute of Health Equity and Public Health England. Available at: www.instituteofhealthequity.org/resources-reports/building-children-and-young-peoples-resilience-in-schools/evidence-review-2-building-childrens-and-young-peoples-resilience-in-schools.pdf

Ankrom, S. (2019) *How Brain Cells Communicate*. Available at: www.verywellmind.com/how-brain-cells-communicate-with-each-other-2584397

Bandura, A. (1998) Health promotion from the perspective of social cognitive theory. *Psychology and Health*, 13(4): 623–49.

Bandura, A., Ross, D. and Ross, S. (1961) Transmission of aggression through imitation of aggressive models. *Journal of Abnormal and Social Psychology*, 63(3): 575–82.

Baumrind, D. (1966) Effects of authoritative parental control on child behaviour. *Child Development*, 37(4): 887–907.

Beattie, A. (1991) *Knowledge and Control in Health Promotion*. Available at: researchgate.net

Becker, M. (1974) The health belief model and sick role behaviour. *Sage Journals*. Available at: https://journals.sagepub.com/doi/10.1177/109019817400200407

Bellis, M. A., Hughes, K., Ford, K., Hardcastle, K. A., Sharp, K. A., Wood, S., Homolova, L. and Davies, A. (2018) Adverse childhood experiences and sources of childhood resilience: a retrospective study of their combined relationships child health and educational attendance. *BMC Public Health*, 18: 792.

Bennett, P. and Murphy, S. (1998) *Psychology and Health Promotion*. Open University Press.

Bennett, C. and Rosner, D. (2019) The Promise of Empathy CHI 2019, May 4–9, 2019, Glasgow. Available at: https://dl.acm.org/doi/pdf/10.1145/3290605.3300528

Berlo, D. (1960) *The Process of Communication: An Introduction to Theory and Practice*. New York: Holt, Reinhart and Winston.

Berry, J. (2016) *Does Health Literacy Matter?* Available at: www.england.nhs.uk/blog/jonathan-berry/

Blumenthal, K., Peter, J., Trubiano, J. and Phillips, E. (2019) Antibiotic allergy. *Lancet* 393(10167): 183–98. doi:10.1016/S0140-6736(18)32218-9

References

Bowlby, J. (1969) *Attachment and Loss: Vol 1. Attachment.* New York: Basic Books.

Bowlby, J. (1977) *The Making and Breaking of Affectional Bonds.* Available at: http://gnakos.ru/wp-content/uploads/2019/10/Making-and-Breaking-of-Affectionate-Bonds-by-Bowlby.pdf

Brandon, M., Sidebotham, P., Belderson, P., Cleaver, H., Dickens, J., Garstang, J., Harris, J., Sorensen, P. and Wate, R. (2020) *Complexity and Challenge: A Triennial Analysis of SCRs 2014–2017.* Department for Education. Available at: https://assets.publishing.service.gov.uk/government/uploads/system/uploads/attachment_data/file/869586/TRIENNIAL_SCR_REPORT_2014_to_2017.pdf

Braungart-Rieker, J. M., Lefever, J. B., Planalp, E. M. and Moore, E. S. (2016) Body mass index at 3 years of age: cascading effects of prenatal maternal depression and mother-infant dynamics. *J Pediatr.*, 177: 128–32. Available at: https://doi.org/10.1016/j.jpeds.2016.06.023

Brownson, R., Baker, T., Deshpande, A. and Gillespie, K. (2017) *Evidence-Based Public Health.* Oxford: Oxford University Press.

Burd, H. and Halsworth, M. (2016) *Making the Change: Behavioural Factors in Person- and Community-Centred Approaches for Health and Wellbeing.* Available at: www.scie.org.uk/prevention/research-practice/getdetailedresultbyid?id=a11G0000009TFkbIAG

Burnard, P. and Gill, P. (2008) *Culture, Communication and Nursing.* London: Pearson.

Cancer Research (2020) *Cervical Cancer Statistics.* Available at: www.cancerresearchuk.org/health-professional/cancer-statistics/statistics-by-cancer-type/cervical-cancer

Chowdary, M. R. (2020) *What Is Coping Theory?* Available at: positivepsychology.com

Cooper, D. (2021) *Report to Health and Social Care Scrutiny Committee.* Bradford Council, February.

Counting Lives (2019) *The Children's Society.* www.childrenssociety.org.uk/sites/default/files/counting-lives-report.pdf

Dahlgren, G. and Whitehead, M. (1991) *Polices and Strategies to Promote Social Equity in Health.* Available at: www.iffs.se/.../policies-and-strategies-to-promote-social-equity-in-health

Davidson, S. (2018) *Age UK Digital Inclusion Evidence Review 2018.* www.ageuk.org.uk/globalassets/age-uk/documents/reports-and-publications/age_uk_digital_inclusion_evidence_review_2018.pdf

Davies, S. (2019) *Time to Solve Childhood Obesity.* Available at: assets.publishing.service.gov.uk/government/uploads/system/uploads/attachment_data/file/837907/cmo-special-report-childhood-obesity-october-2019.pdf

Department of Health (DH) (2012) *Long Term Conditions Compendium of Information,* 3rd edition. Available at: www.gov.uk/government/publications/long-term-conditions-compendium-of-information-third-edition

Department of Health and Social Care (2011) *The Mental Health Strategy for England.* Available at: www.gov.uk/government/publications/the-mental-health-strategy-for-england

Dinh, T. T., Bonner, A., Clark, R., Ramsbotham, J. and Hines, S. (2016) The effectiveness of the teach-back method on adherence and self-management in health education for people with chronic disease: a systematic review. *JBI Database System Rev Implement Rep,* January, 14(1): 210–47. doi: 10.11124/jbisrir-2016-2296. PMID: 26878928

Drucker, P. (1989) *The Practice of Management.* London: Heinemann.

Edwards, N. (2018) Why has the NHS not been copied? Available at: www.nuffieldtrust.org.uk/news-item/why-has-the-nhs-not-been-copied-spoiler-it-has

Ekern, J. (2016) *Effective Coping Skills Used in Eating Disorder Recovery*: Available at: www.eatingdisorderhope.com

Engel, G. (1980) *The Clinical Application of the Biopsychosocial Model.* Available at: https://pubmed.ncbi.nlm.nih.gov/7369396/

Erikson, E. (1950) *Childhood and Society.* W. Norton & Co.

European Union (2018) *EU Data Protection Legislation Article 9.* Available at: www.privacy-regulation.eu/en/article-9-processing-of-special-categories-of-personal-data-GDPR.htm

Farooq, B. (2019) *Self-Harm in Children and Adolescents: Attention Seeking or Cause for Concern?* Available at: www.acamh.org/blog/self-harm-in-children-and-adolescents-attention-seeking-or-cause-for-concern/

Fenton, K. (2017) *A New Focus on Falls Prevention.* Available at: https://publichealthmatters.blog.gov.uk/2017/01/25/a-new-focus-on-falls-prevention/

Francis, R. (2013) *Report of the Mid Staffordshire NHS Foundation Trust Public Enquiry, Executive Summary.* Available at: Report of the Mid Staffordshire NHS Foundation Trust Public Inquiry: Executive Summary HC 947, Session 2012–2013 (publishing.service.gov.uk).

Chartered Society of Physiotherapy (2015) *Get Up and Go: A Guide to Staying Steady.* Available at: www.csp.org.uk/publications/get-go-guide-staying-steady-english-version

Gibson, A. and Asthana, S. (2000) Estimating the socioeconomic characteristics of school populations with the aid of pupil postcodes and small-area census data: an appraisal. *Environment and Planning: Economy and Space,* 32(7): 1267–85. doi:10.1068/a3276

Glasper, A., Coad, J. and Richardson, J. (Eds) (2015) *Children and Young People's Nursing at a Glance.* West Sussex, United Kingdom: John Wiley and Sons.

Gleissner, G. (2017) *Eating Disorders and Stress Eating Disorders and Stress.* Available at: www.psychologytoday.com/england/counselling

Goffman, E. (1963) *Stigma.* London: Penguin.

Golinowska, S. (2016) *Health Promotion Targeting Older People.* Available at: pubmed.ncbi.nlm.nih.gov/27608680 (nih.gov)

Goschin, S., Briggs, J., Blanco-Lutzen, S., Cohen, L. and GalynkerBeth, I. (2013) *Parental Affectionless Control and Suicidality.* New York: Israel Medical Centre NY, Department of Psychiatry.

Government Equalities Office (2018) Available at: https://www.gov.uk/government/organisations/government-equalities-office

Gov.UK (2012, 2021) *NHS Constitution for England.* Available at: www.gov.uk/government/publications/the-nhs-constitution-for-england

Gov.UK (2016) *Childhood Obesity: A Plan for Action.* Available at: www.gov.uk/government/publications/childhood-obesity-a-plan-for-action/childhood-obesity-a-plan-for-action

Gov.UK (2018) Childhood Obesity: A Plan for Action, Chapter 2. Available at: www.gov.uk/government/publications/childhood-obesity-a-plan-for-action-chapter-2

Gov.UK (2020) *Health Inequalities Dashboard.* Available at: www.gov.uk/government/statistics/health-inequalities-dashboard-september-2020-data-update

References

Gov.UK (2021a) *Press Release: New Office for Health Promotion to Drive Improvement of Nation's Health.* Available at: www.gov.uk/government/news/new-office-for-health-promotion-to-drive-improvement-of-nations-health

Gov.UK (2021b) *The Best Start for Life: A Vision for the 1,001 Critical Days.* Available at: https://assets.publishing.service.gov.uk/government/uploads/system/uploads/attachment_data/file/973112/The_best_start_for_life_a_vision_for_the_1_001_critical_days.pdf

Graham, H. (2012) Smoking, stigma and social class. *Journal of Social Policy,* 41(1): 83–99. doi:10.1017/S004727941100033X

Greenfield, J. (2014) *Social Learning Theory and Anorexia.* Available at: www.prezi.com

Guest, J. F., Keating, T. and Gould, D. (2020) Modelling the annual NHS costs and outcomes attributable to healthcare-associated infections in England. *BMJ Open,* 10: e033367. doi: 10.1136/bmjopen-2019-033367

Hagell, A. and Shah, R. (2019) *AYPH Key Data on Young People 2019.* Available at: www.youngpeopleshealth.org.uk/wp-content/uploads/2019/09/Key-Data-on-Young-People-2019-PHE-Conference-Poster.pdf

Hamm, R. M. (1988) *Clinical Intuition and Clinical Analysis: Expertise and the Cognitive Continuum. Professional Judgement: A Reader in Clinical Decision Making.* Cambridge: Cambridge University Press.

Hand Hygiene. Available at: www.england.nhs.uk/wp-content/uploads/2019/03/national-policy-on-hand-hygiene-and-ppe.pdf

Harris, M. (2021) *Understanding Person Centred Care for Nursing Associates.* London: Sage.

Health Education England (HEE) (2016) *Making Every Contact Count (MECC).* Available at: https://www.hee.nhs.uk/our-work/population-health/making-every-contact-count-mecc

Health Education England (HEE) (2017) www.makingeverycontactcount.co.uk/media/27613/mecc-resources-fact-sheet-v9-20180601.pdf

Health Education England (HEE) (2020) *Person-Centred Care.* Available at www.hee.nhs.uk/our-work/person-centred-care

Health Foundation/Marmot Review Ten Years On. Available at: www.health.org.uk/publications/reports/the-marmot-review-10-years-on

Health Matters Making Cervical Screening More Accessible. (2020) Available at: www.gov.uk/government/publications/health-matters-making...

Healthcare Quality Improvement Partnership (HQIP) (2019) *The Learning Disability Mortality Review (LeDeR) Programme, Annual Report.* University of Bristol. Available at: www.hqip.org.uk/wp-content/uploads/2019/05/LeDeR-Annual-Report-Final-21-May-2019.pdf

Hochbaum, G., Rosenstock, I. and Kegels, S. (1952) *Health Belief Model.* United States Public Health Service.

Hogg, S. (2013) *Prevention in Mind: All Babies Count: Spotlight on Perinatal Mental Health NSPCC.* Available at: https://maternalmentalhealthalliance.org/wp-content/uploads/NSPCC-Spotlight-report-on-Perinatal-Mental-Health.pdf

Holland, K. (2019) Understanding the link between alcohol use and depression. *The Alcohol–Depression Connection: Symptoms, Treatment and More.* Available at: www.healthline.com/health/mental-health/alcohol-and-depression

Hopkins, P. (2010) *Young People, Place, and Identity*. London: Routledge.

IGME (2020) *UN Inter-agency Group for Child Mortality Estimation*. Available at: childmortality. org/analysis

Illich, I. (1975) *Medical Nemesis: The Expropriation of Health*. London: Marion Boyars.

Institute for Healthcare Improvement (2021) *SBAR Tool: Situation–Background–Assessment–Recommendation*. Available at: www.ihi.org/resources/Pages/Tools/SBARToolkit.aspx

Institute of Health Equity (2018) *Reducing Health Inequalities through New Models of Care: A Resource for New Care Models*. London: University College London.

Jamison, K. R. In: Crisp, A. H., ed. (2001) *Every Family in the Land: Understanding Prejudice and Discrimination Against People with Mental Illness*. Available at: Stigma.org

Jamoulle, M. and Roland, M. (1995) Quaternary prevention. In: *Hong-Kong Wonca Classification Committee*. Brussels.

Johansen, M. and O'Brien, J. (2015) *Decision Making in Nursing Practice: A Concept Analysis*. New York: Wiley.

Kalkhoran, S., Kruse, G., Chang, Y. and Rigotti, N. (2018) *Smoking-Cessation Efforts by US Adult Smokers with Medical Comorbidities*. Available at: www.amjmed.com/article/S0002-9343(17)31011-2/fulltext

The King's Fund (2015) *Health Inequalities*. Available at: www.kingsfund.org.uk/projects/nhs-in-a-nutshell/health-inequalities

Kmietowicz, G. (2020) *Unvaccinated 'Wakefield Cohorts' Blamed for 5000 Cases of Mumps in England Last Year*. Available at: www.bmj.com/content/368/bmj.m619.full

Leach, P. (2011) *The Essential First Year: What Babies Need Parents to Know*. DK Publishing.

Life Expectancy Statistics. Available at: www.kingsfund.org.uk/publications/what-are-health-inequalities#life

Lindson, N., Klemperer, E., Hong, B., Ordonez-Mena, J. and Aveyard, P. (2019) Smoking reduction interventions for smoking cessation: Cochrane Systematic Review. Available at: www.cochranelibrary.com/cdsr/doi/10.1002/14651858.CD013183.pub2/full

Longley, B. (2020) *Empathy vs Sympathy: What Is the Difference?* Available at: www.thoughtco.com

Madden, A. (2018) *4 Reasons Why You Shouldn't Follow the Latest Diet*. Available at: www.bhf. org.uk/informationsupport/heart-matters-magazine/news/food-trends-2016/do-not-follow-food-trends

Main, M. and Solomon, J. (1990) Procedures for identifying infants as disorganised/disoriented during the Ainsworth Strange Situation. In: Greenberg, M. T., Cicchetti, D. and Cummings, E. M. (eds) *Attachment in the Preschool Years* (pp. 121–160). Chicago, IL: University of Chicago Press.

Marmot, M., Allen, J., Goldblatt, P., Boyce, T., McNeish, D., Grady, M. and Geddes, I. (2010) *Fair Society, Healthy Lives: The Marmot Review. Strategic Review of Health Inequalities in England post-2010*. London: The Marmot Review. Available at: www.instituteofhealthequity.org/resources-reports/fair-society-healthy-lives-the-marmot-review/fair-society-healthy-lives-full-report-pdf.pdf

Marmot, M., Allen, J., Goldblatt, P., Herd, E., and Morrison, J. (2020) *Build Back Fairer: The Covid-19 Marmot Review*. Available at: www.health.org.uk/publications/build-back-fairer-the-Covid-19-marmot-review

References

Marmot, M. J. B. (2020) *Health Equity in England: The Marmot Review 10 Years On*. The Health Foundation.

Maslow, A. (1943) A theory of human motivation. *Psychological Review*, 50(4): 370–96.

May, J., Williams, A., Cloak, P. and Cherry, L. (2020) Still bleeding: the variegated geographies of austerity and food banking in rural England and Wales. *Journal of Rural Studies*, 79: 409–42. Available at: www.sciencedirect.com/science/article/abs/pii/S0743016719308083?via%3Dihub

McLaren, N. (2007) *Humanizing Madness: Psychiatry and the Cognitive Neurosciences*. New York: Future Psychiatry Press.

McShane, M. (2013) *Learning from Those Who Are Doing It*. Available at: www.england.nhs.uk/blog/martin-mcshane-2/

Menon, V., Carrion, V., Duberg, K. and Bostan, S. J. (2020) *Stanford Study Finds Stronger One-Way Fear Signals in Brains of Anxious Kids*. Available at: https://med.stanford.edu/news/all-news/2020/04/stanford-study-finds-stronger-one-way-fear-signals-in-brains-of-.html

Michie, S., van Stralen, M. and West, R. (2011) The behaviour change wheel: a new method for characterising and designing behaviour change interventions. *Implementation. Sci* 6(42). Available at: https://doi.org/10.1186/1748-5908-6-42

Mina, M. J., Metcalf, C., de Swart, R. L., Osterhaus, A. and Grenfell, B. T. (2015) Long-term measles-induced immunomodulation increases overall childhood infectious disease mortality. *Science*, 348(6235): 694–9. doi:10.1126/science.aaa3662

Naidoo, J. and Wills, J. (2016) *Foundations for Health Promotion*, 4th edition. London: Elsevier.

Nadioo, J. and Wills, J. (2020) *Health Promotion: Foundations for Practice* (Public Health and Health Promotion). London: Elsevier.

NHS (2014) *NHS Five Year Forward View*. Available at: www.england.nhs.uk/wp-content/uploads/2014/10/5yfv-web.pdf

NHS (2017) *Five Year Forward View Next Steps*. Available at: www.england.nhs.uk/publication/next-steps-on-the-nhs-five-year-forward-view/

NHS (2019a) *Long Term Plan*. Available at: www.longtermplan.nhs.uk/online-version/

NHS (2019b) *The 5 Steps to Mental Wellbeing*. Available at: www.nhs.uk/conditions/stress-anxiety-depression/improve-mental-wellbeing/

NHS (2020) *Definitions for Health Inequalities*. Available at: www.england.nhs.uk/ltphimenu/definitions-for-health-inequalities/

NHS England (2015) *Communication Cross Cutting Theme for Patient Safety*. Available at: www.england.nhs.uk/signuptosafety/wp-content/uploads/sites/16/2015/09/su2s-comms-safety.pdf

NHS England, Care Quality Commission, Health Education England, Monitor, Public Health England and the Trust Development Authority (2014) *NHS Five Year Forward View*. Available at: www.england.nhs.uk/wp-content/uploads/2014/10/5yfv-web.pdf

NHS Improvement (2021) *SBAR Communication Tool*. Available at: https://improvement.nhs.uk/documents/2162/sbar-communication-tool

NHS@Home. Available at: www.england.nhs.uk/nhs-at-home/

NICE (2014, 2017) *Healthcare-Associated Infections: Prevention and Control in Primary and Community Care*. Available at: www.nice.org.uk/guidance/cg139/chapter/1-guidance

NICE (2015) *Children's Attachment: Attachment in Children and Young People Who Are Adopted from Care, in Care or at High Risk of Going into Care.* NG26. Available at: www.nice.org.uk/guidance/ng26

NICE (2015, 2020) *Antimicrobial Stewardship: Systems and Processes for Effective Antimicrobial Medicine Use.* Available at: www.nice.org.uk/guidance/ng15/resources/antimicrobial-stewardship-systems-and-processes-for-effective-antimicrobial-medicine-use-pdf-1837273110469

NICE (2018) *Post-Traumatic Stress Disorder.* Available at: www.nice.org.uk/guidance/ng116

NICE (2019) *Depression in Children and Young People: Identification and Management.* Available at: www.nice.org.uk/guidance/ng134

NICE (2020a) *Eating Disorders: Recognition and Treatment.* Available at: www.nice.org.uk/guidance/ng69

NICE (2020b) *Making Every Contact Count: How NICE Resources Can Support Local Priorities.* Available at: https://stpsupport.nice.org.uk/mecc/index.html

NICE (2020c) *Sepsis Quality Statement.* Available at: www.nice.org.uk/guidance/qs161/chapter/Quality-statements

NICE (2021) *Informed Consent Guidance.* Available at: www.nice.org.uk/guidance/cg138/chapter/1-guidance

NIH (2021) *Cultural Respect.* Available at: www.nih.gov/institutes-nih/nih-office-director/office-communications-public-liaison/clear-communication/cultural-respect

Nursing and Midwifery Council (NMC) (2018) *Nursing Associate Standards of Proficiency.* Available at: www.nmc.org.uk/globalassets/sitedocuments/education-standards/nursing-associates-proficiency-standards.pd%20f

Nursing and Midwifery Council (NMC) (2020) *NMC Code of Standards.* Available at: www.nmc.org.uk/standards/code/

Nutbeam, D. (2000) Health literacy as a public health goal: a challenge for contemporary health education and communication strategies into the 21st century. *Health Promotion International,* 15(3): 259–67.

Office of National Statistics (2018) *Statistics on Government Healthcare Spending.* Available at: www.ons.gov.uk/peoplepopulationandcommunity/healthandsocialcare/healthcaresystem/bulletins/ukhealthaccounts/2018

Office of National Statistics (2019a) *Child and Infant Mortality in England and Wales: 2019.* Available at: www.ons.gov.uk/peoplepopulationandcommunity/birthsdeathsandmarriages/deaths/bulletins/childhoodinfantandperinatalmortalityinenglandandwales/2019

Office for National Statistics (2019b) *Deaths of Homeless People in England and Wales: 2019 Registrations.* Available at: www.ons.gov.uk/peoplepopulationandcommunity/birthsdeathsandmarriages/deaths/bulletins/deathsofhomelesspeopleinenglandandwales/2019registrations

Office of National Statistics (2020a) *Adult Smoking Habits in the UK: 2019.* Available at: www.ons.gov.uk/peoplepopulationandcommunity/healthandsocialcare/healthandlifeexpectancies/bulletins/adultsmokinghabitsingreatbritain/2019#the-proportion-who-are-current-smokers-in-the-uk-its-consistent-countries-and-local-areas-2011-to-2019

Office of National Statistics (2020b) *Suicide Statistics by Profession.* Available at: www.ons.gov.uk/peoplepopulationandcommunity/birthsdeathsandmarriages/deaths/adhocs/10807suicidebyoccupationenglandandwales2011to2018registrations

References

Office for National Statistics (2021) *Sexual Orientation, UK: 2019.* Available at: www.ons.gov.uk/peoplepopulationandcommunity/culturalidentity/sexuality/bulletins/sexualidentityuk/2019

Ofsted (2018) *Obesity, Healthy Eating and Physical Activity in Primary Schools.* Available at: https://assets.publishing.service.gov.uk/government/uploads/system/uploads/attachment_data/file/726114/Obesity__healthy_eating_and_physical_activity_in_primary_schools_170718.pdf

Ogden, T. and Hagen, K. A. (2019) *Adolescent Mental Health Prevention and Intervention,* 2nd edition. London: Routledge.

Palleja, A., Mikkelsen, K., Forslund, S., Kashani, A., Allin, K., Nielsen, T., Hansen, T., Liang, S., Feng, Q., Zhang, C., Pyl, P., Coelho, L., Yang, H., Wang, J., Typas, A., Nielsen, M., Nielsen, H., Bork, P., Wang, J., Vilsbøll, T., Hansen, T., Knop, F., Arumugam, M. and Pedersen. O. (2018) Recovery of gut microbiota of healthy adults following antibiotic exposure. *Nature Microbiology,* 3(11).

Parsons, T. (1951) *Illness and the Role of the Physician: A Sociological Perspective.* Available at: https://doi.apa.org/doiLanding?doi=10.1111%2Fj.1939-0025.1951.tb00003.x

Pearce, A., Dundas, R., Whitehead, M. and Taylor-Robinson, D. (2019) *Pathways to Inequalities in Child Health.* MRC/CSO Social and Public Health Sciences Unit, University of Glasgow, Glasgow, UK. Available at: https://adc.bmj.com/content/archdischild/early/2019/02/23/archdischild-2018-314808.full.pdf

Peer, R. and Shabir, N. (2018) *Iatrogenesis: A Review on Nature, Extent, and Distribution of Healthcare Hazards.* Available at: www.ncbi.nlm.nih.gov/pmc/articles/PMC6060929/

Pender, N. J., Murdaugh, C. L. and Parsons, M. A. (2011) *Health Promotion in Nursing Practice,* 6th edition. Boston, MA: Pearson.

PHE (Public Health England) (2020) *Community Profiles.* Available at: https://fingertips.phe.org.uk/profile/health-profiles

Pike, S. and Forster, D. (1995) *Health Promotion for All.* Churchill Livingstone.

Positive Behavioural Support Framework (2015) Available at: www.england.nhs.uk/6cs/wp-content/uploads/sites/25/2015/05/pbs-comp-framework.pdf

Price, B. (2017) Developing patient rapport, trust and therapeutic relationships. *Nursing Standard,* 31(50): 52–63. doi: 10.7748/ns.2017.e10909 https://pubmed.ncbi.nlm.nih.gov/28792344

Prochaska, J. and DiClemente, C. (1986) Towards a comprehensive model of change. In: Miller, W. and Heather, N. (eds) *Treating Addictive Behaviours: Processes of Change.* New York: Pergamon.

Public Health England (PHE) (2014) *From Evidence into Action: Opportunities to Protect and Improve the Nation's Health.* Available at: www.gov.uk/government/uploads/system/uploads/attachment_data/file/366852/PHE_Priorities.pdf

Public Health England (PHE) (2015) *Rapid Review to Update Evidence for the Healthy Child Programme 0–5.* Available at: www.gov.uk/government/publications/healthy-child-programme-rapid-review-to-update-evidence

Public Health England (PHE) (2019) *PHE Strategy 2020–25.* Available at: https://assets.publishing.service.gov.uk/government/uploads/system/uploads/attachment_data/file/831562/PHE_Strategy_2020-25.pdf

Public Health England (PHE) (2020) *PHE Live Life Well Portal.* Available at: www.livelifewell.org.uk/

Public Health England (PHE) (2021a) *Start4Life*. Available at: https://campaignresources.phe. gov.uk/resources/campaigns/2-start4life/

Public Health England (PHE) (2021b) *Inclusive and Sustainable Economies: Leaving No-one behind Supporting Place-based Action to Reduce Health Inequalities and Build Back Better.* Available at: www.gov.uk/government/publications/inclusive-and-sustainable-economies-leaving-no-one-behind/inclusive-and-sustainable-economies-leaving-no-one-behind-executive-summary

Public Health England (PHE) (2021c) *School-aged Years High Impact Areas: Supporting Healthy Lifestyles.* Available at: www.gov.uk/government/publications/commissioning-of-public-health-services-for-children/school-aged-years-high-impact-area-3-supporting-healthy-lifestyles

Rabøl, L. I. Andersen, M. L. Østergaard, D. Bjørn, B. Lilja, B. and Mogensen T. (2011) Descriptions of verbal communication errors between staff: an analysis of 84 root cause analysis-reports from Danish hospitals. *BMJ Qual Saf*, March, 20(3): 268–74. doi: 10.1136/bmjqs.2010.040238

Raleigh, V. (2021) *What Is Happening to Life Expectancy in England?* Available at: www. kingsfund.org.uk/publications/whats-happening-life-expectancy-england

Ratna, H. (2019) The importance of effective communication in healthcare practice. *Harvard Public Health Review*, 23. Available at: https://harvardpublichealthreview.org/healthcommunication/

RCN (2019a) *Communication*. Available at: www.rcn.org.uk/clinical-topics/patient-safety-and-human-factors/professional-resources/communication

RCN (2019b) *Health Literacy and Teach Back*. Available at: www.rcn.org.uk/.../health-literacy-and-teach-back

RCN (2021) *Record Keeping*. Available at: www.rcn.org.uk/professional-development/publications/pub-006051

RCPsch (2020) *Two-Fifths of Patients Waiting for Mental Health Treatment Forced to Resort to Emergency or Crisis Services*. Available at: www.rcpsych.ac.uk/news-and-features/latest-news/detail/2020/10/06/two-fifths-of-patients-waiting-for-mental-health-treatment-forced-to-resort-to-emergency-or-crisis-services

Resman, F. (2020) Antimicrobial stewardship programs; a two-part narrative review of step-wise design and issues of controversy Part I: step-wise design of an antimicrobial stewardship program. *Journal of Therapeutic Advances in Infectious Diseases.*

Ritch, D. (1986) Shannon and Weaver: unravelling the paradox of information. *Communication Research*, 13(2): 278–98. doi:10.1177/009365086013002007

Rogers, C. (1961) *On Becoming a Person: A Psychotherapists View of Psychotherapy*. Houghton Mifflin.

Rosen, M. (2020) *These Are the Hands*. Available at: www.scottishpoetrylibrary.org.uk/poem/these-are-hands/

Rowe, G., Ellis, S., Graham, K., Henderson, M., Barnes, J., Counihan, C. and Carter-Bennett, J. (2020) *A Handbook for Nursing Associates and Healthcare Practitioners*. London: Sage.

Royal Osteoporosis Society. Available at: https://theros.org.uk/

Rychter, A. M., Zawada, A., Ratajczak, A., Dobrowolska, A. and Krela-Kaźmierczak, I. (2020) Should patients with obesity be more afraid of Covid-19? *Obesity Review* 21(9). Wiley.

References

Schram, W. (Ed.) (1954) *The Process and Effects of Mass Communication.* Illinois: University of Illinois Press.

Scott, D. and Weston, R. (1998) *Evaluating Health Promotion.* London: Stanley Thornes.

Sense (2016) *Making the Case for Play: Findings of the Sense Public Enquiry into Access to Play Opportunities for Disabled People with Multiple Needs.* Available at: www.sense.org.uk

Shrivastava, A., Johnston, M. and Bureau, Y. (2012) Stigma of Mental Illness-1: Clinical Reflections. *Mens Sana Monogr.,* 10(1): 70–84. doi:10.4103/0973-1229.90181

Sibiya, M. (2018) *Nursing: Effective Communication in Nursing.* Available at: https://books. google.co.uk/books?id=Ib-QDwAAQBAJ&lpg=PP1&pg=PP1#v=onepage&q&f=false

Simon, H. A. (1990) Invariants of human behaviour. *Annual Review of Psychology,* 41(1), 1–20.

Stewart, S. M. and Bond, M. H. (2002) A critical look at parenting research from the mainstream: problems uncovered while adapting Western research to non-Western cultures. *British Journal of Developmental Psychology,* 20(3): 379–92. https://doi.org/10.1348/026151002320620389

Strumpel, C. and Billings, J. (2006) *Overview on Health Promotion for Older People: Report of the European Project 'HealthProElderly'.* Available at: www.healthproelderly.com/pdf/National_report1_Germany_en.pdf

Sun, J., Patel, F., Rose-Jacobs, R., Frank, D., Black, M. and Chilton, M. (2017) Mothers' adverse childhood experiences and their young children's development. *American Journal of Preventative Medicine,* 53(6): 882–91.

Tajfel, H., Turner, J., Austin, W. and Worchel, S. (1979) *An Integrative Theory of Intergroup Conflict. Organizational Identity: A Reader.* Monterey, CA: Brooks and Cole.

Tannahill, A. (1985) What is health promotion? *Health Education Journal,* 44(4): 167–8. Available at: https://journals.sagepub.com/doi/abs/10.1177/001789698504400402

Taylor, S. and Asmundson, G. (2021) Negative attitudes about facemasks during the Covid-19 pandemic: the dual importance of perceived ineffectiveness and psychological reactance. *PLoS ONE,* 16(2): e0246317. https://doi.org/10.1371/journal.pone.024631

Templin, T., Cravo Oliveira Hashiguchi, T., Thomson, B., Dieleman, J. and Bendavid, E. (2019) The overweight and obesity transition from the wealthy to the poor in low- and middle-income countries: a survey of household data from 103 countries. *PLoS Med* 16(11): e1002968. https://doi.org/10.1371/journal.pmed.1002968

Tudor, H. J. (1971) The Inverse Care Law. *Lancet,* 297(7696): 405–12.

Tuovinen, S., Lahti-Pulkkinen, M., Girchenko, P., Heinonen, K., Lahti, J., Reynolds, R. M., Hämäläinen, E., Villa, P. M., Kajantie, E., Laivuori, H. and Raikkonen, K. (2021) Maternal antenatal stress and mental and behavioural disorders in their children. *J Affect Disord.,* 278: 57–65. doi: 10.1016/j.jad.2020.09.063. PMID: 32950844

Walsh, B.T. (2013) The enigmatic persistence of anorexia nervosa: science of eating disorders. *The American Journal of Psychiatry,* 170(5): 477–84. Available at: www.scienceofeds.org/2013/07/07-the-enigmatic-persistance-of-anorexia-nervosa

Watson, M. and Lloyd, J. (2019) *Sure Start Cut Child Admissions and Health Inequalities, Report Finds.* Available at: www.bmj.com/content/365/bmj.l4043/rr

Waugh, A. and Grant, A. (2018) *Ross and Wilson: Anatomy and Physiology in Health and Illness,* 13th edition. London: Churchill Livingstone.

Williams, E., Buck D. and Babalola, G. (2020) What are health inequalities. Available at: www.kingsfund.org.uk/publications/what-are-health-inequalities

World Health Organization (WHO) (1986) *The Ottawa Charter*. Available at: https://www.euro.who.int/__data/assets/pdf_file/0004/129532/Ottawa_Charter.pdf

World Health Organization (WHO) (2010) *Conceptual Framework for Action on the Social Determinants of Health*. Available at: https://www.who.int/sdhconference/resources/ConceptualframeworkforactiononSDH_eng.pdf

World Health Organization (WHO) (2013) *Global Action Plan for the Prevention and Control of Noncommunicable Diseases 2012–2020*. Available at: www.who.int/publications/i/item/9789241506236

World Health Organization (WHO) (2018a) *About Social Determinants of Health*. Available at: www.who.int/gender-equity-rights/understanding/sdh-definition/en/

World Health Organization (WHO) (2018b) *Mental Health: Strengthening Our Response*. Available at: www.who.int/news-room/fact-sheets/detail/mental-health-strengthening-our-response

World Health Organization (WHO) (2018c) *Time to Deliver: Report of the WHO Independent High-Level Commission of Noncommunicable Diseases*. Available at: https://apps.who.int/iris/handle/10665/272710

World Health Organization (WHO) (2018d) *WHO Releases New International Classification of Diseases (ICD 11)*. Available at: www.who.int/news/item/18-06-2018-who-releases-new-international-classification-of-diseases-(icd-11)

World Health Organization (WHO) (2020a) *Health Promotion for Older People: Not Business as Usual*. Available at: www.who.int/ageing/features/health-promotion/en/

World Health Organization (WHO) (2020b) *Social Determinants*. Available at: www.who.int/social_determinants/en/

World Health Organization (WHO) (2021a) *Hand Hygiene*. Available at: www.who.int/campaigns/world-hand-hygiene-day/2021

World Health Organization (WHO) (2021b) *How to Handwash and Handrub*. Available at: https://www.who.int/multi-media/details/how-to-handwash-and-handrub

World Health Organization (WHO) (2021c) *Improving Health Literacy*. Available at: www.who.int/activities/improving-health-literacy

Young, B., Bedford, L., Kendrick, L., Vedhara, K., Robertson, J. F. R. and das Nair, R. (2018) Factors influencing the decision to attend screening for cancer in the UK: a meta-ethnography of qualitative research. *Journal of Public Health*, 40(2): 315–39

Index

Locators in **bold** refer to tables and those in *italics* to figures.